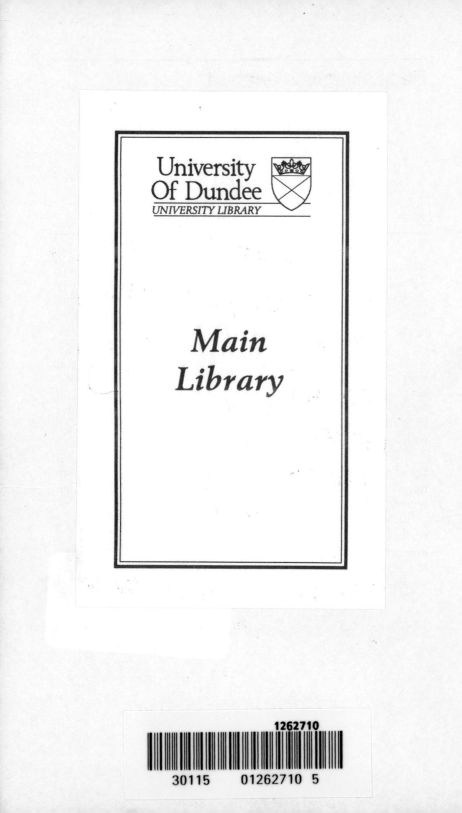

University
Of Dundee
UNIVERSITY LIBRARY

Main
Library

Regulating womanhood

Sexuality, motherhood and marriage were matters of public policy throughout the nineteenth and early twentieth centuries. They were prominent areas in the regulation of women, but the idea that the law merely reflected what was normal and natural obscured the extent of this regulation.

Regulating Womanhood poses historically and culturally specific questions about the mechanisms that have controlled and restricted women. It shows not merely how laws and policies have set boundaries to the lives of women but also how the category of 'woman' has been constructed as a specific object for legal and social policy, and how women came to be seen as needing 'special' regulation.

In addition, *Regulating Womanhood* explores how children and the organisation of reproduction and sexuality operated to normalise and make acceptable the degree of regulation to which women were subjected.

Yet this is not a catalogue of the unmitigated subjection of women in history. The contributors focus on women's resistance and activity, and on the shift in modes of regulation, to challenge the idea of an unchanging history of the legal oppression of women.

Regulating womanhood

Historical essays on marriage, motherhood and sexuality

Edited by
Carol Smart

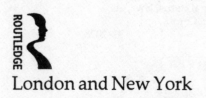

London and New York

First published 1992
by Routledge
11 New Fetter Lane, London EC4P 4EE

Simultaneously published in the USA and Canada
by Routledge
a division of Routledge, Chapman and Hall, Inc.
29 West 35th Street, New York, NY 10001

Typeset from the author's wordprocessing disks by
NWL Editorial Services

Printed and bound in Great Britain by
Mackays of Chatham PLC, Chatham, Kent

British Library Cataloguing in Publication Data
Carol Smart
Regulating womanhood: historical essays on marriage,
motherhood and sexuality.
I. Smart, Carol, 1948–
342.2878

Library of Congress Cataloging in Publication Data
Carol Smart
Regulating womanhood: historical essays on marriage,
motherhood, and sexuality/edited by Carol Smart.
p. cm.
Includes bibliographical references and index.
1. Women – Government policy – History – 19th century.
2. Women – Legal status, laws, etc. – History –
19th century. 3. Women – Government policy – History
– 20th century. 4. Women – Legal status, laws, etc. –
History – 20th century. I. Smart, Carol.
HQ1236.R43 1992 91–20286
305.42'09 – dc20 CIP

ISBN 0–415–06080–X
0–415–07405–3 (pbk)

Contents

Contributors

Lucy Bland is a lecturer in women's studies at the Polytechnic of North London. She has written extensively in the area of British feminism and sexuality in the late-nineteenth and early-twentieth centuries. She is completing a book for the Women's Press to be called *Banishing the Beast: Feminism, Sex and Morality in England, 1885–1918*.

Anna Clark teaches history at the University of North Carolina at Charlotte. She was Fellow of the National Humanities Centre in 1990–91. She is the author of *Women's Silence, Men's Violence: Sexual Assault in England, 1770–1845* (Pandora, 1987), and several articles. Her current project is a book on gender and the making of the British working class. She has also served as a volunteer accompanying battered women to the courts in cases against their husbands.

Carol-Ann Hooper teaches in the Department of Social Policy and Social Work at the University of York, UK. Her main interests are in women and social policy, child care and sexual violence, and she has recently completed research on women's responses to the sexual abuse of their children by other family members. She is the author of several articles on child abuse.

Jane Lewis is a reader in Social Administration at the LSE. She is the author of *The Politics of Motherhood. Child and Maternal Welfare in England, 1900–1939* (1980), *Women in England 1870–1945* (1984), (with Barbara Meredith) *Daughters Who Care* (1988), *Women and Social Action in Victorian and Edwardian England* (1991) and (with David Clark and David Morgan) *Whom God Hath Joined Together: The Work of Marriage Guidance, 1920–1990* (1991).

Selma Sevenhuijsen is a political theorist and Professor of Interdisciplinary Women's Studies at the University of Utrecht. She was formerly lecturer in political theory and history at the University of Amsterdam. She has written in the fields of women and the state, motherhood and reproductive politics, the family and its history, feminist political theory and feminism and ethics. Her publications include *Child Custody and the Politics of Gender* (edited with Carol Smart) 1989 and *Equality Politics and Gender* (edited with Elizabeth Meehan) 1991.

Martine Spensky is a lecturer in the Department of English Studies and participates in the Women's Studies Module of the University of Paris VIII. She is also responsible for the research group 'Social Policies and the State in European Countries' in the same university. Her publications include 'Les bourgeoises anglaises interdites de travail au dix-neuvième siècle', (1990) in *Les Cahiers de Charles V*, Université de Paris VII and 'Les mères célibataires dans l'Angleterre Thatchérienne: les effets du *Social Security Act* de 1986 sur cette population', in *Les Cahiers de l'Observatoire*, special issue on 'Pauvreté et Assistance', 1990, no. 2, June, Université de Clermont-Ferrand.

Carol Smart is Professor of Sociology at Leeds University and formerly senior lecturer in sociology and women's studies at the University of Warwick, UK. She has been Distinguished Visiting Professor at Osgoode Hall Law School, York University, Toronto and the Belle van Zuylen Visiting Chair in the School of Women's Studies at Utrecht University. She has written exten- sively in the field of feminism and law. Her recent publications include *Feminism and the Power of Law* (Routledge, 1989) and *Child Custody and the Politics of Gender* (edited with Selma Sevenhuijsen, Routledge, 1989).

Mariana Valverde teaches social theory and feminist issues in the Sociology Department at York University in Toronto, Canada. Her main research interests lie in the history of moral regulation in Canada and in Britain. Her most recent book is *The Age of Light, Soap, and Water: Moral Reform in English Canada 1880s–1920s* (Toronto, McClelland & Stewart, 1991).

Ursula Vogel is lecturer in political theory at the University of Manchester. She has written extensively on women in classical political theory and has research interests in the fields of citizenship, the history of liberalism, the Enlightenment and Romanticism. She has recently published *The Frontiers of Citizenship* (edited with M. Moran, Macmillan, 1991) and is currently writing a book on property rights and power in marriage.

Introduction

Carol Smart

This edited collection is part of an ongoing project whose main aim is to continue to refine and develop feminist 'legal' scholarship. I have put 'legal' in quotation marks because the book takes law and legality in its widest sense, and all the contributors approach their specific subjects from a social history/social scientific perspective rather than a strictly legal one. The book is also a theoretical enterprise as much as an historical exercise. Whilst I am not assuming that historiography is a theory-free exercise, the papers in this collection are addressed to, or imbued with, concerns over current theoretical debates about the construction of the category 'Woman', the various forms of theoretical and political dissent with feminism itself and the ways in which social regulation is productive of both subjects (of regulation) and of resistance. These theoretical concerns are pursued through some very detailed analyses of specific historical moments and/or debates occurring mostly in late-nineteenth or early-twentieth-century Britain.

The specific focus is modes of regulation through sexuality, marriage and motherhood. However, the book as a whole does not treat these as discrete entities but works to show how they interrelate to create a specifically gendered form of social regulation. A most important sub-theme is the linkage of women and children and the development of discourses on motherhood and caring as productive of forms of gentle, and not so gentle, regulation. It would seem to be increasingly the case that we cannot understand the workings of forms of regulation without giving some degree of priority to how the category of Woman is constructed in relation to the category of the Child.

Since the early contribution by Dahl and Snare (1978) on the coercion of privacy, feminist legal scholarship has been interested in informal, private, virtually invisible forms of regulation not acknowledged as such in mainstream criminology or sociology of law. This interest was paralleled in wider feminist scholarship by a concern with analysing the family. Indeed it became a powerful tenet of feminist theory that women's oppression originated in the family. In this collection we are not seeking to resurrect this argument but, because of the critique of much feminist work on the family which has emerged in the last 10 years, it is perhaps necessary to say why the so-called private sphere remains an important site of investigation.

Feminist theoretical work has recently been the subject of considerable intellectual struggle. I am not referring to divisions between different 'schools' like radical feminism, socialist feminism and so on, so much as to modes of theorising. Much second-wave theorising was oriented to finding answers to the BIG questions of women's oppression, to marrying marxism and feminism or theories of capitalism and patriarchy, and to making sweeping statements as to the origins of oppression. This tendency remains, and indeed remains attractive in many ways. However, another discernible trend has emerged and that is the tendency to abandon grand theorising in favour of more detailed, small-scale, historically specific analyses which are much more sensitive to differences between women rather than constructing women as a monolithic, homogeneous category in opposition to other categories like men, class or 'race'. In coming to grips with differences based on class, 'race', religion and/or region, feminist theory has also had to begin to accede to the idea of differences amongst women.

Grand theorising, for all its promise of a fundamental answer to women's oppression, is incapable of dealing with difference in a sufficiently subtle or detailed way. Moreover, it seems wedded to giving priority to one form of oppression over others in the last instance if not the first. Feminist work has begun to appreciate that we cannot add class and 'race' to a pre-eminent category of women and hope to do justice to the specificity of the production of classed, 'raced' and gendered subjects.

In consequence, the focus on what might be regarded as the family or at least the private in this collection is not a revival of a general claim that therein we can find the source of the oppression of all women. On the contrary, the chapters remain located within the theoretical boundaries of the specific and do not seek to make sweeping statements. But I am not in any case convinced that we should assume that issues of sexuality, motherhood and reproduction really do exist within the private sphere. As these chapters show, from the mid-nineteenth century at least, they become matters of public policy and concern. The point that is made here is more that the definition of certain behaviours as private is part of the regulatory impulse which has a specifically gendered set of consequences.

Another major sub-theme in this collection is the project to recapture aspects of women's resistance to and participation in events which regulate women. This book sees itself as in opposition to that project (if it is still ongoing) which seeks to depict women as the victims of patriarchy or patriarchy's law. We do not therefore add documentation to the story of the endless grinding of women, nor do we seek to show how patriarchy develops more and more cunning modes of oppression. Rather, our intention is to acknowledge women as cultural agents where this is warranted. We hope also to avoid that other oversimplification of pointing to women's 'complicity' in women's oppression by being cautious of too many value judgements based on a feminist perspective developed in the late twentieth century.

The chapters that follow are grouped thematically rather than chronologically, with the first chapters dealing mostly with aspects of sexuality and reproduction in conjunction with forms of regulation developed within philanthropy and social work. The later chapters take as their focus aspects of marriage, the marriage relationship and its legal consequences.

The first chapter by Carol Smart seeks to map out aspects of the theoretical debate which is based upon the argument that legal discourses are constitutive of the subject 'woman', not simply a mode of control imposed on independent or simply 'given' individuals. It seeks to explore how the different feminine subjects of law are constituted in classed and 'raced' as well as gendered terms. This is pursued through an analysis of specific legislation concerning sexuality and motherhood in the late nineteenth century. Lucy Bland (Chapter 2) builds on this by focusing on the role of feminist campaigners and reformers in the field of vice and sexual exploitation at the end of the century. Central to this chapter is the idea of women as cultural agents and the development of competing feminist strategies in relation to the use of law. A key issue is the thorny problem of the slippage of protection into repression of which nineteenth-century feminists were well aware.

Carol-Ann Hooper's chapter (Chapter 3) should be read in conjunction with Bland's because it continues these themes but in the field of child sexual abuse. Central to Hooper's thesis is the construction of child sexual abuse in relation to motherhood in early philanthropic discourse. Changing definitions of childhood led to the surveillance of mothers, not fathers, and Hooper explores this paradox. She concludes that responses to child sexual abuse were designed to protect an ideal of motherhood rather than to regulate fathers.

Hooper's chapter concludes with a discussion of contemporary social work, and this is followed by Jane Lewis's detailed analysis of the development of social work in the late nineteenth century (Chapter 4). Lewis is critical of the 'women controlling women' model that has developed in the field of social work and criminal justice and seeks to differentiate between the work carried out by early middle-class women social workers and the development of social work policy which was dominated by men and the state. She does not suggest that there was only one strategy developed by the early feminist social workers, however, and her chapter explores some of these theoretical and political differences.

Spensky continues the focus on social work practice and theory in Chapter 5 but in the context of law on illegitimacy and unmarried motherhood. She examines the rise of mother-and-baby homes and the theoretical justifications for denying or pathologising unmarried motherhood as a form of motherhood and for imposing a system of adoption on young mothers. For Spensky, the rise of the mother-and-baby home is analysed in a way similar to the rise of the asylum or the prison, in other words as a disciplinary regime which sought to 'normalise' this form of deviance.

The central issue in Mariana Valverde's chapter (Chapter 6) is a case study of the Dionne quintuplets who became popular icons of idealised childhood in Canada in the 1930s. Her focus is the construction of childhood rather than motherhood, and this particular case reveals the contradictions that existed in state policy concerning children. The Quints (as they became known) were simultaneously idealised childhood (subjected to the most modern scientific methods of childrearing) and 'non-children' (revenue-generating tourist attractions). This moment in history is a fascinating 'blip' in the development of theories of the welfare of the child and reveals the power associated with abstract fatherhood rather than practical mothering.

With Ursula Vogel's chapter (Chapter 7) we turn more directly to the issue of marriage and sexuality, specifically the question of adultery and the double standard of morality. Vogel compares developments in two different legal traditions, the common law tradition of England and the civil code tradition of Germany at the end of the last century. She challenges the idea of an unchanging imposition of a static, patriarchal norm by revealing the specific historical, legal and economic factors involved in the waxing and waning of the use of the double standard in law. She argues, for example, that the paradox of liberalising the divorce law was the imposition of a rigid double standard which was not formerly given such priority. Her argument also details how wives' adultery moved from being a matter of private control to one of public (state) regulation.

In Chapter 8 Selma Sevenhuijsen analyses the development of concepts of citizenship which were so central to liberal thought in the nineteenth century but points to the way in which competing evolutionary theories located women in the private sphere of the family, thus denying them the public benefits associated with the concept of citizenship. Citizenship was male, and as long as women were primarily constructed as mothers they could not 'fit' into the emancipatory movements of the period. Sevenhuijsen points to the fear of autonomous women which developed at the same time as the first-wave women's movement in Europe. This gave rise, however, to the paradox of women being granted the status of citizens in public law, long before these rights were conceded to them in private (family) law.

The final chapter is by Anna Clark, who deals with a slightly earlier period in British legal history, namely the late-eighteenth and early-nineteenth centuries. Her focus is the issue of wifebeating and the inadequate response of law to this form of violence. Her argument is, however, that although we can witness a sorry history of neglect of women, we can see women using and making demands of the legal system throughout these periods. Where the police failed to help women they would resort directly to the magistrates courts, and Clark points to the irony that, as the state took on a more 'protective' role towards women, they actually lost the important autonomy of being able to prosecute cases themselves. Clark uses the distinction offered by Carole Pateman between the social contract and the sexual contract, showing how the social contract did not extend protection from violence to married women (although it did to women victims of stranger assault), whilst the sexual contract legitimated the abuse of women in marriage.

Together, these chapters seek to make a contribution on a number of levels. They bring together new historical material, new theoretical insights and new visions of women as social agents who negotiate law and related forms of control rather than simply being its victims. There are no 'answers' to be found here, but the book will have succeeded if it challenges unreflexive or over-simplified statements on the relationship between 'women' and 'law', and adds to our understanding of how mechanisms of regulation have become transformed into taken-for-granted routines in social work and legal theory and practice.

ACKNOWLEDGEMENTS

I am grateful to the resources and facilities of Osgoode Hall Law School at York University, Toronto, where I was Distinguished Visiting Professor during the editing of this book. Special thanks are due to Eva Heilimo for all her valuable secretarial assistance and skill.

Chapter 1

Disruptive bodies and unruly sex
The regulation of reproduction and sexuality in the nineteenth century

Carol Smart

INTRODUCTION

In this chapter I wish to explore certain modes of regulation which effectively construct a specific category of 'Woman' whilst seeking to contain the problematic Woman thus constructed. My focus is therefore on discursive constructs/subjects and the complex ways in which discourses of law, medicine and social science interweave to bring into being the problematic feminine subject who is constantly in need of surveillance and regulation. A key focus is the dominant idea of disruption and unruliness which is seen to stem from the very biology of the body of Woman.

I am not seeking to use an analysis which might promise to reveal the real woman beneath an historically specific patriarchal veneer. Neither am I attempting to distinguish myth from reality, or truth from falsehood. This is not, of course, to say that 'real' women have not existed historically. Rather, it is to suggest, following Riley (1988), that the category of Woman is constantly subject to differing constructions. Woman is not a singular unity that has existed unchanged throughout history as certain feminist, religious and biological discourses might proclaim. Rather, each discourse brings its own Woman into being and proclaims her to be natural Woman.

But unless it now sounds as if I am arguing that women are mere plastic, the quintessential cultural dupes of history, let me emphasise that there have always been multiplicities of resistance against such constructions. Not only have there always been contradictory discursive constructs of Woman at any one time, thus allowing Woman herself to be contradictory, but the subject, Woman, is not merely subjugated; she has practised the agency of constructing her subjectivity as well. So Woman is not merely a category, she is also a subjective positioning within which there is room for manoeuvre.

My focus here, therefore, is the construction of Woman in legal discourse; a Woman who is simultaneously brought into being and subjected to specific modes of regulation because of characteristics designated as natural within the discursive act of her very construction. My point is that, whereas many women experienced the modes of regulation thus imposed, not all feminine subjectivity was necessarily coterminous with the Woman in the discourse. I am seeking to explore how legal, medical and early social scientific discourses intertwine to produce a woman who is fundamentally a problematic and unruly body; whose sexual and reproductive capacities need constant surveillance and regulation because of the threat that this supposedly 'natural' woman would otherwise pose to the moral and social order. At the same time I am not presuming that the forms of regulation imposed are always (or even often) 'successful' in the sense of achieving a modified subjectivity or even moderated behaviour. The former is a question which can probably never be resolved if we are looking at historical subjects; the latter is more open to scrutiny but that would be a different project to the one undertaken in this chapter.

If we accept that even dominant discursive constructions of Woman may vary, we meet the possibility of a range of contradictions within this categorisation. Women were thus constructed as both powerful and powerless, as sexual agents but also as victims, as dangerous but in need of protection. This is not a new insight but it is perhaps time for us to go beyond remarking this apparent set of contradictions to try to understand in greater detail how they were manifested and able to persist. I think we can only do this if we take seriously a poststructuralist theory of power and a deconstructionist view of the category woman. Let us start with the latter issue; an approach which is the project of Butler's *Gender Trouble* (1990). As she states:

> As a genealogy of gender ontology, this inquiry seeks to understand the discursive production of the plausibility of that binary relation [between the real/authentic and the illusory/ artificial] and to suggest that certain cultural configurations of gender take the place of 'the real' and consolidate and augment their hegemony through that felicitous self-naturalization.
>
> (Butler 1990: 32–3)

She is therefore concerned to explore how certain constructions of gender occupy the cultural space known as the 'real' or the 'natural'. Once we begin to understand gender in these terms we move beyond a debate which claims authenticity for the Woman constructed by a specific discourse. We must also be cautious about how we utilise the notion of 'contradictions' when we discover the wide variety of discursive constructions of gender. The very term contradiction can suggest an ideological conflict capable of resolution by reference to the 'real'. The idea that Woman is both powerful and powerless, sexual victim and sexual agent and so on is uncomfortable for a feminism that has invested much in its own construction of Woman as powerless and victimised. Within feminism we have therefore tended to resolve the political and conceptual problems posed by the recognition of these 'contradictions' by separating them out. By this I mean that we have argued, for example, that white women are powerful when compared to black women, but are powerless when compared to white men. We have created a kind of role theory to accommodate these apparent contradictions, so that we can understand their manifestation in sociospacial or economic terms. In doing this we have operated with a concept of power as a material possession which is held or withheld as we move from one situation to another. This conceptual device has meant that feminist theory has continued to construct its pre-eminent category Woman, but when this 'univocal posturing' is challenged, feminist discourse has relied upon sociological strategies to avoid the criticism that its conceptualisation is oppressive. By this I mean that when this construct, Woman, is challenged, we have simply sought to add class and gender as *variables* but at a completely different level of conceptualisation. Thus class and race, and we might add religion, are prefixed to the dominant theoretical categorisation. Hence we have working-class women, black women, muslim women. This formulation, of course, retains the underlying assumption that they are all Woman, that their 'Womanness' is held fast in some way. We have only to think of the introduction of terms like 'lady doctor' or 'woman lawyer' to see how deeply problematic this linguistic and sociological device is. It is not so much a solution as a masking of the problem.

This line of argument is made forcibly by Spelman (1988) who argues that many attempts to add class and race to gender have merely obscured or reflected racism and classism. Because of the additive approach we have conceptually segregated and hence continued the fragmentation of bodies begun by imperialist, eugenicist, classist and sexist discourses. This is not to say that there have not been political gains made by 'disavowed categories' who have re-evaluated their class, race, gender or 'disability', but as Spelman has argued such advances have often incurred the exclusion of other categories. Indeed, this becomes transparent when we rephrase some fairly well-established political slogans, for example, 'A (white, middle-class, Protestant) Woman's Right to Choose'. Again, this may not be a new insight, but the question remains one of how to respond to such important critiques.

I have suggested that the 'listing of variables' approach is problematic for political and theoretical reasons. As Riley has tersely stated, 'Below the newly pluralized surfaces, the old problems still linger' (Riley, 1988: 99). I want also to add that it is inadequate at the level of theory for epistemological reasons. Put simply it takes for granted that there are unproblematic empirical factors that must now be theoretically processed. Harding (1986) has pointed to the inadequacy of feminist empiricism which adds the variable Woman, and then stirs. The same point must be made in relation to this extended form of empiricism. The task that is required is not to add, but to reconceptualise. We have to re-do feminist theorising.

This is, of course, easier said than done. Many feminist theorists are now looking to poststructuralism as a way of reconceptualising (Hekman, 1990; Butler, 1990; Weedon, 1987). As bell hooks (hooks, 1990) has argued, however, to date the decentred subject and fragmented subjectivities of this mode of theorising have not attracted much interest amongst black scholars. Postmodernism looks white. But it does offer to deconstruct whiteness; the question is whether this 'offer' will be taken up. It has certainly begun the process of challenging the 'univocal posturing of the regulatory fictions of sex and gender' (Butler, 1990) whether these posturings are from within feminist discourse or not.

There are no clear guidelines for reformulating feminist theory, but certain forms of historical analysis offers us the chance to deconstruct Woman, not just in terms of gender, but also in terms of class and race. In other words we can look to the specificity of certain gendered, classed and raced constructs and avoid the seductive trap of generalising or fundamentalising (i.e. arguing that one element is the fundamental oppression) that has become a feature of standpoint theorising and/or grand theorising. As Valverde has argued:

> The Marxist–feminist debates on the relationship between capitalism and patriarchy, for example, which absorbed so much energy in the seventies, have in many quarters now given way to: (a) concrete analyses of how class, gender and race actually interact and (b) a poststructuralist rejection of 'models' in favour of an examination of shifting meanings. It is symptomatic that some of the most innovative feminist research done today consists precisely of a combination of social history and post-structuralist method.
>
> (Valverde, 1990: 63)

This project is therefore fundamental to this chapter. That is to say I wish to consider the specific conditions of the production of the Woman of legal discourse in one historical period without presuming a 'univocal posturing'.

THE HISTORICAL CONTEXT

My focus is the period between 1860 and 1890. This is a particularly significant period in Victorian Britain because of the rise of legislation oriented towards social engineering. While the principles of Common Law dominated in all legal spheres, the nineteenth century as a whole (but with increasing pace towards the end and into the twentieth century), introduced more and more sophisticated legislation for enactment. Behaviours apparently requiring regulation became more precisely specified, or it might conversely be argued, were partly brought into being by campaigning rhetoric and legal prohibitions. As various technologies developed, the law could become more precise. Hence legislation governing the incarceration of prostitutes under the Contagious Diseases Acts of 1866 and 1869 was influenced by medical advice as to how long it took to cure venereal diseases. The implementation on legislation governing infanticide was dependent upon forms of medical knowledge which claimed to differentiate between the baby who had breathed on birth and the one who had not and was, therefore, technically stillborn.

Law, either in the form of new legislation or in the form of more effective enforcement of established legislation, marched hand in hand with medical science. Indeed, even a cursory glance at the witnesses called to give evidence to Parliamentary Select Committees on topics like 'white slavery', prostitution and the preservation of infant life, shows the growing influence of the medical profession on legal developments. But medical science and even lay elements involved in moulding law for social engineering purposes, were reliant on yet another form of scientific activity. This was the science of social investigation and statistics. Basic statistics on births, deaths and marriages began to be collected in the early nineteenth century. By the latter half of the century trends became discernable. Put another way, this scientific discourse produced a new subject amenable to regulation, namely populations. Only once statistics on infanticide, abortion, infant mortality and so on became available, could both the pressure for reform be exercised and the necessary precision for specifying culprits and victims be deployed. A good example of this process is the campaign to introduce a criminal law against incest in England and Wales at the end of the nineteenth century. While medical arguments on the problems of interbreeding were relevant, it was not until statistics became 'available' as to the extent of incest that Parliament relented and made incest a criminal offence in 1908.

Foucault (1979) has identified this process as one in which the principle of right (traditional law and authority) engages with the principle of normalisation (the impulse towards correctionalism in its widest sense), which in turn becomes part of the transition to a disciplinary society. As has been pointed out on many occasions, his genealogy of this period does not specifically incorporate the significance of gender to this process. This is made up for in part by the work of Donzelot (1979) but we still have a long way to go before we can understand how gender differentiation operates in the spheres of discipline and punishment. Meanings attributed to the female/feminine body and the male/masculine body are obviously relevant here. So, for example, the extent to which the woman's body is seen as susceptible to unruly impulses, or the extent to which the man's body is deemed to be transcended by his capacity for rational thought might indicate the progress or regress of the disciplinary impulse in different spheres of regulation. This analysis is necessary not to 'prove' that women are more susceptible to more regulation than men, but in order to understand how gender 'works' (see Poovey, 1989).

I shall start with a consideration of how law as discourse constructs the unruly feminine body. I shall then consider how medical and social sciences contributed a new dimension to this unruliness and how law sought to transform the unruly body into the docile body. Central to these constructions of Woman as body are, of course, her sexuality and reproductive capacities.

CONSTRUCTING THE UNRULY FEMININE: LEGAL DISCOURSE

'Why, at this specific historical period, should women have been perceived as being in possession of a disruptive sexuality that needed to be disciplined and controlled?' (Shuttleworth, 1990: 54). Shuttleworth is speaking of the Victorian epoch in which medical discourse and popular advertisements sought to construct woman as unstable because of her menstrual cycles and reproductive capacities. Law had sought to regulate women's sexuality and reproduction long before this period, but the last half of the nineteenth century marks a specific moment of struggle over the use of law to regulate the feminine body. It is during this period that we find a surge of legislative and juridical activity concerning sexual and reproductive behaviour. I shall draw upon the following:

(a) 1861 Offences Against the Person Act
(b) 1866 and 1869 Contagious Diseases Acts
(c) 1872 Infant Life Preservation Act
(d) 1885 Criminal Law Amendment Act

In addition I shall draw upon the trial and execution in 1870 of Margaret Waters, who ran a baby-farming business, and the trials of Annie Besant in 1877 and 1878, the first concerning the publication of information on birth control, and the second concerning the loss of custody of her daughter.

These measures reveal an intense legal gaze on issues of reproduction, mothering and sexuality. The 1861 Offences Against the Person Act contained clauses which dealt with rape, procuring, carnal knowledge, abortion, concealment of birth and exposing children to danger. The Contagious Diseases Acts imposed a form of sanitary incarceration on working-class women who became registered as prostitutes in and around garrison towns. The Infant Life Preservation Act concerned baby farming and the practices of working-class mothers who could not care for their children because of employment outside the home. Finally, the Criminal Law Amendment Act was concerned with the so-called White Slave Trade and the procurement of English girls for foreign brothels. It also dealt with brothels at home, other forms of sexual exploitation of underage girls and it raised the age of consent to 16. There are, of course, other examples of this intensity of gaze. For example, the 1857 Matrimonial Causes Act which introduced secular divorce, focused extensive attention on the harm occasioned by a wife's adultery and the need for husbands to have access to divorce in such cases. (The husband's adultery was seen in quite a different light, see Vogel, Chapter 7, this volume.) However, these particular legislative measures and infamous trials, are linked to moments of intense concern, often taking the form of moral panics over the threat that certain behaviours were deemed to be posing to a stable social order.

Not all of these instances deployed the same discursive constructs of sexuality and mothering but the figure which recurs throughout is both the product of her nature (viz physiology) and yet a danger to the natural order (viz social order). The mother who farms out her baby, takes an abortifacient, smothers her infant at birth is not the idealised mother of much Victorian literature. But equally the mother who farms out her infants etc. is constructed in terms of a rhetoric of class rather than one of sexual difference. The prostitute or fallen woman on the other hand, is constructed in terms of the frailty of femininity or by reference to the immorality/sexuality/woman nexus. It is therefore useful to consider the kind of argumentation drawn upon in these different legal manifestations.

In connection with the construction of categories of class, 'race' and sex in the nineteenth century, De Groot has argued that:

> Whereas the theories and practices related to 'class' distinctions and relationships were founded on the new 'sciences' of political economy and social investigation, theories and practices related to 'race' and 'sex' drew on biological, anthropological, and medical scholarship, often grounding themselves in part on observable and 'inescapable' physical aspects of difference.
>
> (De Groot, 1989: 92–3)

This is a useful formulation in that it begins to clarify what otherwise can look like a confusing array of accounts. By extending this idea we can see that in some instances Woman is treated as a 'class issue', while in others as a 'sex issue' or a 'race issue'. By this I mean that primacy is given to certain factors in direct relation to the explanatory paradigm that is invoked. What is being suggested here is that Woman is not only constructed in discourses which address themselves explicitly to sexual difference. Woman can be constructed through theories of class and race and not merely through theories of sex and gender. Unless we can begin to appreciate this more fully, we can never escape the additive model criticised above.

De Groot therefore takes us forward with her analysis of representations of 'sex' and 'race'. But we need to make this model still more complex because we can now understand that even the construction of specific notions of sexual difference are linked to ideas about racial difference and class difference. So De Groot's argument that theories of class drew upon one set of discourses, while theories of 'race' and 'sex' drew on another, does not capture the extent to which class is gendered, sex is 'raced' and so on. For example, Sinha's (1987) work on white masculinity and imperialism shows the linkages between quite specific forms of racism (against Indian men) and an association between proper (white) masculinity and sexual restraint (at least where very young women were concerned). Equally, Davin's (1978) work on British motherhood and imperialism has shown the importance of ideas of racial superiority to specific practices of motherhood. We need therefore to have a multilayered conceptualisation rather than a linear or discreet form of model building. But as Valverde (1990) has argued, this is best achieved through an analysis of a specific historical issue.

REPRODUCTIVE ACTS

In this section I shall look closely at aspects of infanticide, abortion, birth control and baby farming. These activities are the reverse side of the coin of motherhood and perhaps not surprisingly became political and legal issues at a moment when motherhood was being redefined and increasingly confined to a specific model of caring activity (Davin, 1978; Donzelot, 1979; Lewis, 1980). Each of these activities became an affront to the ideal of motherhood at specific moments in the late-nineteenth century.

Infanticide

At common law, infanticide was no different to the murder of adults but an Act passed in 1623 in the reign of James I cast the killing of illegitimate children in a different light. This Act put the burden of proof of innocence on the unmarried mother of a dead infant rather than the more usual practice of placing the burden of proving guilt on the state. The Act is interesting, not only in its extreme harshness (the punishment was hanging), but in the way that it specified bastard children as special victims. This specific focus on illegitimate children and hence unmarried mothers remained a feature of legislation dealing with concealment of birth until 1828 and with infanticide until 1861, but in practice unmarried mothers were constructed as the prime suspects for child murder for rather longer than this.

This Act of James I was repealed in 1803. It was by then well known that juries refused to convict women accused of this crime and so the burden of proof was shifted back to embrace a presumption of innocence. In addition, a new offence was created, namely concealment of birth, which carried a penalty of 2 years' imprisonment. There was, however, a sort of double jeopardy involved in these offences because, if a woman was acquitted on a charge of murder because of lack of evidence, she could still be found guilty of the lesser charge of concealment. The 1803 Act was later consolidated into the Offences Against the Person Act 1961. Additional deterrents were added, however, because it was made a crime for anyone (not just the mother) to conceal a birth whether the infant was born dead *or* alive.

Infanticide therefore has a long legal history but it became a matter of considerable concern between 1860 and 1865 (Behlmer, 1979). Statistics on infant mortality had begun to indicate an increase in infanticide and more accounts became available of the discovery of infant bodies in alleys and woods. The supposed practice of killing babies was regarded as a sign of moral decline, and infanticide in Britain became identified with practices of female infanticide recently discovered in the subcontinent of India (Behlmer, 1979: 407). The crime was therefore seen as a heathen act, one propagated by peoples not fully civilised or human (see Pinkerton, 1898). The person who could commit such an act is therefore already constructed as immoral and un-British.

Yet, there is another important issue which should be included here. This was the role of the medical profession (especially coroners who were drawn from the profession) in translating a variety of infant deaths into infant murder. The growth of medical technologies which created finer categories of causes of death were fundamental to this process. But individual members of the medical profession also cast themselves in the role of moral entrepreneurs in the process of re-evaluating infant life. Drawing upon powerful discourses of medical science and social statistics, combined with a melodramatic narrative genre in which to describe the deaths of innocents, infanticide became redefined as a threat to the social order and civilised values.

We have, therefore, a kind of paradox. At the time of James I in 1623 the laws against infanticide were draconian, thus suggesting a high evaluation of infant life. However, the fact that only unmarried mothers were subject to this law suggests that the focus was less the infant than the sexual and reproductive behaviour of a woman who had no man to support her. Moreover, it would seem that juries understood the economics of infanticide. Without support single women simply could not keep themselves and their infants alive. This relationship between infanticide and poverty was revealed most clearly during 1834 and 1844 when changes to the Poor Law made it virtually impossible for unsupported mothers to find financial relief. During that period infanticide rates rose considerably (Sauer, 1978). There grew, however, a tension between these traditional economic 'understandings' of infanticide and modern medical 'understandings' which increasingly attributed infanticide to puerperal insanity and various disturbances which occurred periodically in women's bodies.

Laqueur (1987) has developed this latter point in considerable detail, pointing out how the nineteenth century gave rise to quite distinct 'understandings' of women's unstable and unruly reproductive functions. The whole metaphor of women's bodies became one of instability of womb and mind. The criminal trial, moreover, became a forum for the public expression and consolidation of such constructions of the feminine. (Another nineteenth-century example would be the rise of kleptomania, see

Abelson, 1989.) We can see, therefore, the extent to which explanations based on economic understandings began to give way to those based on medical ones. But there was never a complete transition and both construction can be said to coexist.

Abortion

It would seem that rates of infanticide began to decline towards the end of the nineteenth century, but as they did concern grew over abortion. At Common Law, abortion after quickening had always been an offence although it would seem that before 1800 no one had ever been convicted of it (Sauer, 1978). In 1803 the first criminal statute against abortion was introduced and it criminalised abortion at any stage of pregnancy, but distinguished between those periods before and after quickening by imposing different levels of punishment. A number of small amendments were made to this Act in 1828, 1837 and 1861. These amendments gradually equalised the punishment for abortion such that there was no distinction between stages of pregnancy. But most importantly the 1861 Act (Offences Against the Person) made the pregnant woman herself the main focus of concern. Prior to this the law was drafted in such a way that those administering poisons etc. to a woman were liable to prosecution, the woman herself was an accessory. The shift is not insignificant in that the earlier legislation takes as its focus a 'profession' or potential 'profession' which might seek to provide the means for a woman to terminate a pregnancy. By the end of the nineteenth century, the pregnant woman herself became the main villain and the need to find the supplier of the poison or device could be dispensed with for the sake of a prosecution.

So, abortion was treated gradually more seriously and more women found themselves enmeshed in the criminal law. This, however, coincided with the historical moment when abortion started to become (relatively) safer and less physically traumatic because of developments in medical technologies. The decline in infanticide would seem to be linked to the increased availability of safer abortions and the increase in the numbers of prosecutions for abortion seem linked in turn to the extent to which women were beginning to favour terminations over neglectful or active infanticide.

The growing concern over women availing themselves of abortions was less amenable to explanations in terms of physiologically induced insanity than was the concern over infanticide. To a large extent it remained within framings of class and poverty. However, such explanations were challenged when married women turned to abortion as well. These women fitted more readily into the category of unnatural mothers who wished to thwart their natural role and the purpose of marriage. Only much later did the single mother become categorised in similar terms (see Spensky, Chapter 5, this volume).

Birth control

It is in the area of birth control that rather different modes of analysis become apparent. Infanticide and abortion were seen as the means deployed by poor working-class women to regulate reproduction and pressures upon them to conform were less concerned with the value of the lost offspring than with a struggle over who should control unruly populations. The practice of birth control was seen as a different kind of threat, at least initially, because the decline in the birth rate from the 1880s was regarded as problematic for the quality of the population. It was feared that the poor were overproducing and the higher classes were failing to replace themselves. This fear was set not only in an eugenicist context but also an imperialist one in which there was a fear that the white races would be overrun by those of 'lesser value'. Foucault (1981) refers to the construction of the Malthusian couple as part of the deployment of power *vis à vis* populations. More accurate might be a focus on the mother or potential mother as a key actor in the struggle over this form of regulation. The point is that men/fathers were rarely invoked in nineteenth-century debates over birth control. They may have been called upon to lessen the sufferings of their wives, and in practice methods of contraception such as withdrawal, rhythm and the condom required their active co-operation. Yet the issue was a woman's issue. It was women, rather than men, who were to be denied the knowledge of the various methods and it was women rather than men who were constructed as 'unnatural' or a threat to the moral order if they engaged in such practices.

McLaren (1978) has pointed to the competing interests involved in the struggle over birth control in the nineteenth century and, following his analysis, it is by no means clear that all women were in favour of birth control. Equally important, the medical profession at this time was not interested in supporting birth control, and the mainstream of the profession disassociated itself from the movement in the early stages. Indeed, the public face of the profession presented contraceptive methods and devices as injurious to health.

The main obstacle to the spread of knowledge of contraception was, however, the fear of unleashing female sexuality and the fear that marriage would be undermined by the subversion of its main purpose (i.e. biological reproduction). Birth-control methods, therefore, had to be rendered dangerous by the detractors, whilst the promoters aimed to 'domesticate' them, that is to make them safe, pro-family and familiar. The struggle to redefine birth control was particularly hard for Victorian women who, in promoting contraception, became associated with all the immoral values attached to the practice itself. Just as it was hard for many suffragists to become involved in issues of prostitution because of the taint of immorality, so too was there considerable risk in being involved in campaigns for contraception.

The trials of Annie Besant in 1877 and 1878 capture this process. The first trial was a prosecution for obscene libel brought against her and Charles Bradlaugh for republishing an American pamphlet by a Dr Knowlton, entitled *Fruits of Philosophy; or, the Private Companion of Young Married Couples* at the price of 6 pence. The trial was a showpiece rather than a run-of-the-mill prosecution. Besant and Bradlaugh had republished the pamphlet precisely to challenge the informal censorship that was operating in relation to the dissemination of this kind of knowledge. But it was also a show trial in as much as both defended themselves in person and were able to put before the court, and hence the public, articulate arguments on sexuality, marriage and contraceptive practices.

What is particularly interesting about Besant's speech is the sources of knowledge she draws upon. She used Malthus, Darwin and social statistics to mount a case against traditional Christian morality. Her argument was pro-marriage and pro-sex but it was based on an idea of ordination by Nature rather than God. Moreover, for her what was ordained by Nature was discoverable through scientific method. She stated:

I can show you from Mr Darwin – that what Knowlton says about health is shown to be true by the fact that married women live longer than unmarried women, and this is a point you get right through every census table that you can take up. You will find there that marriage has a distinctly lengthening effect on human life; you will find that bachelorhood or spinsterhood distinctly shortens life; and it is only reasonable it should be so, gentlemen, because those who despise the natural instincts of nature can scarcely be surprised if nature revenges herself by shortening the life which they do not know how to use. I will put it to you . . . that unmarried women . . . suffer from a number of diseases, special to the reproductive organs, that married women, as a rule, do not suffer from, because they have not thwarted nature in the fashion that those who lead a celibate life must do.

(Besant, quoted in Manvell, 1976: 85–6)

Besant went on to argue that marriage was not only naturally ordained, but that early marriage, coupled with contraceptive practices to reduce the size of families, would solve problems of immorality and prostitution and the exploitation of young working-class women.

What is revealing about Besant's speech is the extent to which she accepts a particular notion of Woman as constructed in scientific discourses and attempts to use this version as if it were a form of emancipatory knowledge. Unfortunately for her, it was precisely the espousal of such views which 1 year later lost her the custody of her 8-year-old daughter to her estranged husband. Whilst the judge in the obscene libel case had obviously been impressed by Mrs Besant's intelligence and loquacity, the judge in the custody case found her an unfit mother precisely because of this sign of unorthodoxy.

Although Besant was ultimately acquitted (on a technicality) on the charge of obscene libel, and she later published her own work on birth control, the movement did not become widely influential until after the trial of Marie Stopes in the 1920s. She had attempted to harness theories about women's nature to a pro-woman cause, but these theories were not free-floating evident truths but discourses which made the intelligent, speaking woman (i.e. Besant herself) an oxymoron. Once moved to the arena of a custody battle in which she was judged in terms of mothering, the self-same intelligent articulateness quickly disqualified her. Mothers could not be free thinkers; mothers follow their maternal instincts.

Baby farming

We have so far considered three moments of reproductive behaviour. Each of these can be seen in terms of means and devices whereby women could detach themselves from children in a context where legal policy sought to keep them fairly firmly attached. Baby farming was another means of achieving detachment. Although baby farming took a number of forms, around 1870 a considerable moral panic arose about the form which virtually guaranteed the permanent demise of many of the infants farmed out. In these cases some working-class women set up businesses which offered to take care of babies for a small amount each week, but then neglected them, or kept them in such deprived conditions that they failed to thrive.

In 1870 Margaret Waters was tried, found guilty and hanged for causing the death of at least four children in her charge (Pearsall, 1975). She was almost certainly the tip of a much larger iceberg as Pearsall argues that the Sunday newspapers were full of advertisements by baby farmers charging minimal rates for the care they provided. Waters had been discovered by a policeman posing as a father who had found nine infants in a very malnourished state in her charge. Other cases also came to light at this time and concern was generated in a vein similar to the virtual moral panic over infanticide. In this instance, however, the villain was not the mother but the 'professional' carer/disposer of children. Notwithstanding this, the debates that followed were preoccupied with issues of motherhood and poverty as much as with restricting baby farming. In 1871 a Select Committee of the House of Lords was set up to consider what should be done. The main reasons they offered for the existence of baby farming were the shame and poverty of the unmarried mother, the inability to care properly for the child, lack of support from the putative father and the limited means of the mother. All of these reasons coincide with the reasons known to contribute to infanticide and abortion. In other words this form of dangerous motherhood was constructed in class terms.

Following the Select Committee's Report, an Act for the Protection of Infant Life was introduced in 1872. This set up a system to license and regulate childminders. It set certain standards for the care of infants, standards which were not extended to public institutions like the workhouse. Such measures should be seen as precursors to the later development of health visitors and methods of 'training' working-class women for motherhood (Davin, 1978; Lewis, 1980). Moreover, what is significant about this Act and the whole tenor of the Select Committee Report is that although it moves towards licensing and surveillance, rather than simply criminal sanction, it remains entirely silent on the central problem facing working-class women of how to earn a living and look after children. By the early twentieth century, mothers who try to do both are clearly being defined as bad mothers (Martin, 1911) but in 1870 the value of the child had not been so much redefined as to bring about prosecutions of mothers for neglect (other than neglect that caused death or serious injury).

The 1872 Act and the subsequent amendment Act in 1897 were part of a process that tried to establish certain standards for mothering. Legislation and/or prosecutions dealing with infanticide, abortion and birth control were more about establishing the fact of motherhood, rather than its quality. The relationship between law and the social and medical sciences is central to these developments and we can see how motherhood is rendered more and more inevitable – at least for working-class women. I have argued elsewhere (Smart, 1982) that legal restrictions on divorce only really became onerous to ordinary women once state-regulated and recorded marriages were required after 1752. The possibility of informal marriage had the benefit of informal divorce. Once all marriage was formalised, legal penalties could be secured to those who tried to leave marriages. Similarly, with the specific construction of motherhood during the nineteenth century it became more difficult for working-class women to avoid 'keeping' their babies. This in turn coincided with a high point in the historic condemnation of unmarried motherhood and bastardy. This, I would argue, makes it clear that the struggle of meaning that was going on was not simply about revaluing infants and children, it was about the construction of a specific form of motherhood which disqualified working-class women from participation in public life. But at the same time we can witness the construction of poor women as dangerous mothers in legal discourse. With the development of more and more of this 'philanthropic' legislation/regulation we can begin to understand the extent to which the whole system of modern social work is founded upon a classed construction of inadequate mothering which is now so taken for granted that the idea of its historical construction is almost regarded as specious.

Thus far we have considered the extent to which, in De Groot's (1989) terms, theories of political economy and social investigation and theories based on medical and biological scholarship have competed and/or co-operated in the production of a specific notion of motherhood and hence Woman. It is usually observed that the latter part of the nineteenth century marks a struggle between working-class life and middle-class values. However, it may be fruitful to develop this idea somewhat differently. Putting it simply, when understood in class terms, acts such as infanticide, abortion, contraception and baby farming are rational responses to severe legal and material penalties consequent upon unmarried motherhood at times of virtual persecution. The dangerous mother is therefore contained within the working classes or the immoral classes. However, the rising influence of the medical profession loosened these boundaries because such acts became less associated with economic conditions and more associated with an instability or dangerousness inherent in the body of all women. What is also apparent is the extent to which marriage as a formal legal status, locates women inside or outside certain categories of dangerousness. The unmarried mother was the most dangerous of all, not only to her infant but also to the social order. The married mother, on the other hand, existed within a restrictive system of tutelage which gave her husband almost complete governance over her should she become a threat. In this sense she may have been a private problem, but she was not generally constructed as a public one. In becoming public problems, as with the cases of married women like Caroline Norton and Annie Besant, the courts simply removed their children from them and they effectively ceased to be mothers. In consequence, we cannot really talk about women without reference to marriage any more than we can talk about women apart from class and other differences. Marriage was a major signifier in the process of constructing the meaning of Woman in legal discourse in the latter part of the nineteenth century.

SEXUAL ACTS

If marriage, after the Marriage Act of 1752, became a systematic mode of regulating the dangers of instability (private and public) posed by the potential unruliness of women's bodies, it is possible to argue that there would be an almost irresistible impulsion towards providing the regulation that marriage promised in cases where women were outside the ties of matrimony. The state gradually became a sort of moral husband through the development of forms of 'protective' legislation.

But what becomes even clearer in this sphere than in the sphere of reproduction is the overarching significance of 'race' to the concepts of protection and sexual morality. In the nineteenth century the concept of sexual morality is clearly white. Those who fail to achieve this standard are less than white; less than British. Hence, not only were colonised peoples seen as less moral, but so were Continental Europeans, the French and the Belgiums being particularly suspect. In this way I think we can begin to understand that sexual morality was not only constructed along gender lines; men of other 'races' were as suspect as working-class women at home. Indeed, we can see a distinct tension between the protectionist moves of the 1861 Offences Against the Person Act and the 1885 Criminal Law Amendment Act and those in the Contagious Diseases Acts of 1866 and 1869. The former were apparently concerned with protecting women (British women against foreign men, young women against old men) whilst the latter was about protecting men of all classes from working-class women. We have therefore a number of quite subtle boundaries being established as part of the extension of regulation over sexuality/ies. Licit sex is not merely defined as that between married (heterosexual) couples, but between people within acceptable age brackets, of acceptable 'races' and doing only acceptable things.

It is of course questionable whether legislation which aims to protect ultimately has this function or whether it further establishes procedures of surveillance and regulation (Gorham, 1978; Hooper, Chapter 3, this volume). The 1861 Act, for example, established 12 years as the age of consent for young women as a means of protecting them against sexual exploitation. However, it can be forcefully argued that rather than providing protection (since the legislation has only ever been used in very specific cases) it constructed young women as incapable of sexual responsibility.

It was part of a process of defining Woman in relation to body and bodily impulses which, whilst not a new strategy in and of itself, was new in relation to the development of law in the field of sexuality. Boys were specifically excluded from this measure even though they too might have been defined as children and open to exploitation under the age of 12. The consequences of this process are described thus by Spelman:

> [W]oman has been portrayed as essentially a bodily being, and this image has been used to deny her full status as a human being wherever and whenever mental activity as over against bodily activity has been thought to be the most human activity of all.
>
> (Spelman, 1982: 123)

The concern for the abduction of heiresses, which predates the 1861 Act can, towards the end of the nineteenth century, be seen to be transformed slowly into a specific concern about sexual activity in general rather than a concern specifically about property. By 1885 this is further developed. The age of consent is raised to 16 years. The first part of the Act, which was originally entitled *The Suppression of Prostitution*, was retitled during the Parliamentary debate to be referred to as *The Protection of Women and Girls*. This section reiterated much of the existing law on procurement but extended it to cover the removal of young women abroad (i.e. the so-called white slave trade). It also brought parents into the criminal justice frame by introducing prosecutions against parents or other guardians who colluded with the procurement. Brothels in England and Wales also came under much tighter control leading to considerable hardship for many women forced on to the streets (see Bland, Chapter 2, this volume).

The campaign leading up to the 1885 Act has been much discussed and the role of the moral panic induced by the journalist W.T. Stead and the *Pall Mall Gazette* is well known (Bristow, 1977; Weeks, 1989). We are also familiar with the extent to which many women involved in prostitution were resistant to the increasingly dominant construction of themselves as innocent victims who only wanted help to return to a virtuous life (Walkowitz, 1984). Such an image was presented by Alfred Dyer, a publisher who was active in a range of vigilance campaigns, when he gave evidence to the House of Lords Select Committee on the Law Relating to the

Protection of Young Girls in 1881. He offered the classic Victorian
vignette of the wronged, innocent young woman whom he helped
to escape from a brothel in Brussels. His story was full of distaste
for the Belgian authorities who refused to help him save this
young woman. The Belgian police were constructed as corrupt and
uncaring, and the 'foreign' system of licit brothels was regarded as
appalling. However, his evidence should be compared with
accounts by British officials and police who were much more likely
to see the women themselves as blameworthy, ungrateful and
reluctant to return to England given the opportunity.

On the other hand, the mothers of these young women were
also held responsible. A Mr Vincent, Director of Criminal Investigations in London, stated in evidence that:

> There are houses in London . . . where there are people who will
> procure children for the purposes of immorality and prostitu-
> tion, without any difficulty whatsoever above the age of 13,
> children without number at 14, 15 and 16 years of age. . . . Now
> it constantly happens, and I believe in the generality of cases it
> is so, that these children live at home; this prostitution actually
> takes place with the knowledge and connivance of the mother
> and to the profit of the household.
>
> (Evidence to the House of Lords Select Committee,
> 19 July, 1881: 63)

Evidence such as this explains why the 1885 Act introduced
sanctions against mothers and these measures can be seen as an
extension to the forms of disciplining working-class motherhood
introduced in 1872 and in various other measures dealing with
children.

It is also clear from the evidence given by the police that
prostitution was regarded by them as a problem of public order
with which they had insufficient powers to deal. This construction
of the police as a thin blue line against the forces of moral disorder
was not a new theme. In 1885 it was to the fore because the
Government had promised to repeal the Contagious Diseases Acts.
Although these never applied to London or other civilian towns, it
was obvious that the police were anxious about their authority on
the streets. Indeed many of those campaigning for the repeal of the
Contagious Diseases Acts saw the 1885 Act as a means of
continuing the harassment of working-class women.

This view of the police as holding back tides of immorality was also paramount earlier in the nineteenth century. Nead (1988) has argued that prostitution and policing became a major issue in 1857 which was a moment of crisis for the Empire. She argues:

> At this moment in the history of imperialism, definition of empire and definitions of morality were intricately interwoven; during a period of imperial crisis the danger and fear could be realized in terms of social and sexual behaviour and, conversely, regulation of sexuality could be articulated in relation to its effects on nation and empire. Questions of military needs, empire and colonial trade could easily be reframed as issues of morality, health and national strength. The moral panic set the stage for the legal regulation of sexuality and the re-definition of class, race and gender.
>
> (Nead, 1988: 84)

Rhetoric about cleaning vice off the streets was imbued with the ideas of extending Christian morality to immoral peoples all over the world. Cleaning up the domestic front became part of the same imperative as that of preserving empire.

Clearly, the Contagious Diseases Acts were part of this imperative. Moreover, in 1869 when the original measures were extended there was a clear feeling that they were 'working'. The Proceedings of the Select Committee on the Contagious Diseases Acts in July 1869 stated that 'Prostitution appears to have diminished, its worst features to have been softened, and its physical evils abated' (p. 2). Indeed, so keen was the Committee on the benefits of the Act that it recommended that the next Parliamentary Session spend time considering extending it to the whole civilian population.

The most obvious villain constructed by this legislation was the lascivious working-class woman who could undermine the health of the nation both directly and indirectly. Yet while the threat of immorality and disease was constructed through metaphors linked to preserving the Empire, the disease itself (like AIDS a century later) was 'raced'. That is to say the medical men called to give evidence to the Select Committee referred to 'imported syphilis' as being the main problem and the venereal disease most resistant to treatment. The woman not only spread disease, but foreign disease.

At a time when ideas about women's sexual anaesthesia were at their height (Cott, 1979) it became imperative to regulate unruly sexuality which had become perceived of as both natural (basely instinctual) and unnatural (the result of moral deprivation). The main strategy used was the criminal law, which sought to punish visible signs of offence. This was complemented by philanthropic work which sought the redomesticisation of apparently eroticised women. Both of these strategies reinforced the boundaries of acceptable behaviour at the symbolic level. They also sexualised and fetishised women's bodies at precisely the same moment that strategies concerning enforced motherhood were being refined. What is important, therefore, is to consider how these two elements interweave. Foucault (1981) hints at this in his description of the process of 'hysterization' of women's bodies. He sees this as a threefold process whereby women's bodies became saturated with sex, then pathologised/medicalised and then given the biologico-moral responsibility of Motherhood. Through this process the Mother, with her negative doppelganger the Nervous Woman, is created.

Insightful though this is, it does not really help us to understand the multilayering of strategies which coexist at any one time. By this I mean that this process derives from an understanding of the specific historical location of bourgeois women in the Victorian era. Whilst, for example, we might agree that women's bodies in general were saturated with sexuality, it is not clear to me that this has the same meaning for all heterogeneous communities of women. But here I am in danger of slipping into the 'variables' approach I was critical of to start with. Would Foucault be more useful if we could add 'race' and 'class'? A more useful approach might be to work with his schema in a more precise way than he was able to do in his brief introductory volume to his incomplete work on sexuality.

Foucault argues that from the eighteenth century we can observe the emergence of the deployment of sexuality. This strategy builds upon the deployment of alliance. The latter is a system of rules governing sexual relations in which the central issue is the formation of linkages between families and the circulation of wealth. It is based on negative sanctions, laws of marriage, legitimacy and inheritance. By contrast, the deployment of sexuality is linked to the economy through the body which produces and consumes, however the power it exercises is more amorphous, more flexible and more extensive. It engenders new objects of control and new means of exercising control rather than relying on rules which seek to fix relationships in a static way. Now, according to Foucault, the deployment of sexuality has not replaced the deployment of alliance, although it might eventually do so. What is interesting in this for the analysis here is that we can see quite clearly how this struggle unfolds differentially for different groups of women. The latter part of the nineteenth century gave rise, I would argue, to a renewed version of the deployment of alliance where poor women were concerned. The move towards enforced motherhood brought with it an emphasis, necessarily, on marriage. Attaching children to women was a way of attaching women to marriage and the whole set of legal statuses that flowed from it. And, even though the circulation of wealth was not an issue for poor women, the structures of the New Poor Law benefit system meant that marriage could be essential for survival for single mothers (see Spensky, Chapter 5, this volume). We might speak, therefore, of a revival of the deployment of alliance affecting working-class women, and giving rise to class- and gender-specific modes of regulation.

Notwithstanding this, we can see some signs of the way in which the deployment of sexuality was beginning to operate. Laws promoting the 'protection' of girls built on and extended the whole idea of confessing sexual irregularities. Women were called upon to tell their stories of seduction and entrapment, and then to tell how they were saved. But in general I would argue that the deployment of sexuality was not a form of regulation affecting working-class women until well into the twentieth century. Rather, we can see the extension of negative sanctions, informed and even mediated by the medical and new social sciences, which sought to impose a very rigid grid of control on the newly observed problem of unruly women of the 'lower orders'.

CONCLUDING REMARKS: REGULATING THE UNRULY BODY

I argued in the introduction that the discourses of law, combined with medicine and social science, brought into being a problematic feminine subject who, at the moment of her constitution, 'self-evidently' required regulation. In other words she always already required some sort of surveillance, regulation or tutelage. The power of these constructs is precisely in the element of 'felicitous self-naturalization' raised by Butler (1990: 33). Thus, the term prostitute always already confirms associations between class, immorality and disease and the need for police and public health intervention. Equally, the concept of motherhood implies the terms and conditions under which mothering is deemed appropriate. All of these elements are assumed to follow naturally. What we have seen, however, is that this process of self-naturalisation is a stark struggle over meaning rather than the smooth emergence of the inevitable. What becomes taken for granted has been contested, and is open to renewed contestation albeit that it is exceedingly difficult to challenge the seemingly self-evident.

The construction of women's bodies as unruly and as a continual source of potential disruption to the social order has given rise to more and more sophisticated and flexible mechanisms for imposing restraint and achieving desired docility. Yet, we must be cautious of recreating a conspiracy theory of history or assuming an unwavering chain of developments further to subjugate women. The point is that the desired docility is not always forthcoming as the continuing struggles over abortion, contraception, childcare and sexuality testify. But what these continuing engagements also testify to is the extent to which women remain constituted in bodily terms. The consequences of this are not always negative, but in the field of law there is a very negative heritage to deal with. Contemporary versions of these nineteenth-century issues, for example, the introduction of evidence on premenstrual tension into criminal trials or the more general assertions of mind/body instability (Allen, 1987) or the incarceration of women who have broken the 'gender contract' by failing to marry or have children (Carlen, 1983) all transport us into a field of understanding in which women are always already problematic. It matters not whether one is arguing that PMT should or should not be allowed in; what matters is the way in which women are already framed by the very legitimacy of asking such a question.

The negative association of Woman/Body apparent in law (especially criminal law) should not lead us to assume that we must repudiate or deny the body in preference for the mind/rationality formulation as some early feminists did (Spelman, 1982). It is this duality itself which is problematic and which forms a kind of trap for the unwary. The problem is that each reference to the gendered (hence feminine) body implies the superiority of the ungendered (hence male) mind. We need, therefore, to do far more to understand how specific gendered, classed and raced meanings have been built into our understandings of the body and how the feminine continues to invoke a regulatory impulse which seems so self-evidently natural.

ACKNOWLEDGEMENTS

I am grateful to Karen Thompson-Harry who was my research assistant at Osgoode Hall Law School where I began the preliminary research for this chapter.

Chapter 2

Feminist vigilantes of late-Victorian England

Lucy Bland

In 1894, two American male guests of social purity feminist Mrs Laura Ormiston Chant complained to her that on their recent visit to the Empire Theatre of Varieties, a large and famous music hall in Leicester Square, they 'were continuously accosted and solicited by women and . . . very much shocked by the want of clothing in the ballet'. In autumn of that year, along with Mrs Hicks, national organiser for the British Women's Temperance Association, Mrs Chant set off for the Empire music hall to establish the veracity of their claims. Bonnetted and in smart but 'discreet' evening dress, she was determined not to stand out as an outsider, a 'prying prude'; in an earlier visit, her 'day' dress betrayed her as other than a regular patron of the music hall – 'I was a marked woman' (Chant, 1894a). Her disguise did not stretch to the wearing of décolletage, however: 'No one has carried on a more consistent campaign against the normal style of evening dress than I have. Ever since I was 21 I have abjured bare neck and arms' (Chant, 1895).

She was appalled by what she witnessed. Not only were some of the performers revealing too much flesh, but worst of all, prostitutes were present in the audience – or rather, in the auditorium, since they were not strictly a *part* of the audience. According to Mrs Chant, they were not there to watch the performances; they came to watch for potential clients. *The Vigilance Record* related her account of the visit:

> The women complained of were very much painted and more or less gorgeously dressed; they did not go into the stalls; they either sat on the lounges or sofas, or took up positions on the top of the stairs, and watched particularly the men who came up to the promenade. In no case were these women accompanied

by gentlemen, or by any others, except of their own type. She noticed a middle-aged woman who introduced the others to a number of gentlemen. . . . The attendants appeared to be on very friendly terms with many of the women.

(*The Vigilance Record*, October 1894)

By this she was implying that the 'Empire' knew well enough the intentions of these women – they were regulars and part of the music hall's attraction.

On 10 October 1894 Mrs Chant was present when the London County Council (LCC) Licensing Committee met to consider applications for the renewal of music hall licences. Licensing of London's approximately 400 music halls, a function formerly held by magistrates, had passed to the Council on its inauguration as administrator of London under the 1888 Local Government Act. Mrs Chant was attending the Licensing Committee in order to challenge the renewal of the Empire's licence, on grounds of indecency on the stage and disorderliness in the auditorium. Although bent on eliminating 'demoralizing' entertainment, Mrs Chant was at pains to stress that she was not against amusement *per se*. Although a member of the National Vigilance Association (hereafter NVA), a social purity organisation, she insisted: 'I am no Puritan' (Chant, 1894a). 'We don't want to lessen the amusements . . . but we will have them decent. They will not be as highways of ruin to the young, licensed opportunities for the vicious' (Chant, 1895). By 'decent' Mrs Chant meant entertainment which was 'respectable' and family-centred, so that 'the husband could take his wife there without the fear that they would be confronted with the slave of the libertine and the keeper of questionable houses' (Chant, 1894b).

Not all feminists applauded Mrs Chant's actions. Josephine Butler, for example, informed a close friend:

I tried hard to keep out of the 'Empire' conflict . . . I continue to protest that I do not believe that any real reform will ever be reached by outward repression . . . [L]et individuals alone, not . . . pursue them with any outward punishment, nor drive them out of any place, so long as they behave decently.

(Butler, 1894, personal letter)

A 'repressive' response to moral matters from *feminists* was of particular concern to Josephine Butler; it had been troubling her for several years. A number of feminists, once apparently *laissez-faire* and anti-statist in matters of sexuality and morality, were now, in the 1880s and 1890s, adopting a more 'repressive' stance and were taking to closing brothels, clearing the streets of prostitutes and attempting to 'clean up' indecent leisure pursuits, from literature to music halls. Why were these women acting in this way?

THE CRIMINAL LAW AMENDMENT ACT 1885 AND THE NVA

The 1880s was a period of low profit, high unemployment, severe cyclical depression and a chronic housing shortage. This economic instability combined with political developments – the rise of socialism and the immigration into the East End of London of foreign anarchists – to generate a deep fear amongst the propertied classes of a working-class uprising (see Stedman Jones, 1976). But it was not just overtly political beliefs and activities which were seen as a threat; immoral behaviour, too, was viewed as potentially subversive. Further, the desire for moral reform was present even in the pursuit of what might appear to us today as predominantly *material* reform. For example, the concern to improve working-class housing partly related to the belief that overcrowding encouraged incest and juvenile prostitution (Stedman Jones, 1976: 224).

Through legislation and philanthropy, many efforts were made to encourage the working class into a middle-class 'decency'. While the respectable working classes were wooed, the casual poor – the 'dangerous classes' – were policed more coercively, and their behaviour, including their leisure pursuits, was subjected to greater intervention. All this may give us a small part of the explanation for the interventionist activities of certain middle-class feminists, but it is clearly not enough. For a greater understanding of their actions, it is important to look, amongst other things, at the changing relationship of women to public space, women's role within philanthropy and local government and ideas concerning female sexuality. But first, what exactly was this 'repressive' activity in which a number of feminists were now engaging?

The story of this apparent volte-face needs to start earlier, in the 1870s. Throughout the 1870s, Josephine Butler's energy was directed towards the abolition of the Contagious Diseases (hereafter CD) Acts. The legislation had been introduced in the 1860s to regulate prostitution in the hope of countering venereal disease amongst the army and the navy. The Acts introduced into certain military depots the forced inspection, detention and treatment of women who were suspected of being prostitutes. By the 1870s, opposition to the Acts had sprung up in the form of a coalition of middle-class evangelicals, working-class radicals and an active group of feminists headed by Butler. Despite the difficulties entailed in such diverse groups attempting to work together, sufficient numbers of MPs had been converted to the repeal cause to win suspension of the CD Acts in 1883.

In 1885, after 15 years of fighting for the abolition of the Acts, there was much optimism that their repeal was close at hand. In her address to a meeting in the spring of that year, Josephine Butler spoke of a new concern, namely the 'repressionists' in their midst: those bent on abolishing prostitution and introducing moral behaviour through repression. At this point, however, she was adamant that:

> these people are not our enemies ... mistaken as we think they are in their methods, [they] are still honestly desirous of getting rid of prostitution; ... the advocates of the Contagious Diseases Acts desire the very opposite. They believe prostitution to be a necessity. ... It is the fervent desire of my heart to win and gain over entirely to our side all that crowd of repressionists who are now ... going in a distinctly wrong direction, but who may be won.
> (Butler, 1885, *The Shield*, 11 April)

The CD Acts were repealed in 1886. A year later, Butler's concern with repressive actions remained. It was now voiced specifically in relation to Britain's central social purity organisation, the National Vigilance Association, which at this time numbered many repealers amongst its members, Josephine Butler included, although her membership was merely nominal (*The Sentinel*, April 1887). It provided support to victims in cases of sexual assault and rape, including the offer of a solicitor's services. It argued for the introduction of women magistrates and women police, and campaigned to change various aspects of the law concerning sexual offences (see Jeffreys, 1985). Butler praised the NVA's involvement in these activities; her unease lay primarily with another aspect of its work – its attempts to enforce certain clauses of the Criminal Law Amendment Act concerning brothels.

Butler was not alone in her concern. Veteran feminist and repealer Elizabeth Wolstenholme Elmy was similarly worried about 'those with whom for 17 years I have worked for the Repeal of the Contagious Diseases Acts', who, 'by a strange perversion, now sanction and command the means and the methods of a cruel repression' (Wolstenholme Elmy, May 1887). Mrs Chant was one such example, a member of both the feminist repeal organisation, the Ladies National Association and the NVA. Ten years later, having lost hope long ago of winning over such people, Butler warned her colleagues:

> Beware of 'Purity Societies' . . . ready to accept and endorse any amount of inequality in the laws, any amount of coercive and degrading treatment of their fellow creatures in the fatuous belief that you can oblige human beings to be moral by *force*, and in so doing . . . promote social purity.

(Butler, 1897)

It was still the NVA to whom she was principally referring.

The NVA had been set up by social purists in order to ensure the enforcement of the Criminal Law Amendment Act of 1885. The Act had hurriedly passed through Parliament in the wake of W.T. Stead's sensationalist 'revelations' in the *Pall Mall Gazette* in July of that year on the extent of London's juvenile and coerced prostitution. There had been unsuccessful attempts to secure a Criminal Law Amendment Bill for a couple of years, each Bill aiming to raise the age of consent and reform the law on sexual assault. Most feminists supported these measures, but the Bills also contained various repressive clauses relating to soliciting and brothels. The Vigilance Association for the Defence of Personal Rights (known since its beginnings simply as the 'Vigilance Association') of which Josephine Butler and many other repealers had been founder members in 1871, had always been wary of each new version of the Bill. Despite its chief aim being opposition to 'over-legislation' in the name of personal freedom, it gave guarded support to the version of the bill which finally got through. (Incidentally, it made no reference to the clause which criminalised 'indecent acts' between men.) Its journal commented: 'The clauses giving increased irresponsible power to the police in the streets have been struck out, and the other clauses . . . have been so altered that the power of the police is less, while that of the public is greater.' Nevertheless, it warned that:

> a law however just, must be justly and wisely administered. . . .
> In the present case there is far more than the usual amount of
> probability that mischief may be done, on account of the
> formation . . . of voluntary associations to put the law in motion,
> and the difficulty of ensuring . . . that they shall always act with
> prudence and justice.
>
> (*The Journal of the Vigilance Association*, 15 October 1885)

Most of such voluntary associations affiliated themselves to the
NVA. The Vigilance Association for the Defence of Personal Rights
was also far from happy with the NVA's choice of title. Since the
NVA had 'filched from us our good name' (ibid), the following year
the Vigilance Association changed its own to the 'Personal Rights
Association'.

The Vigilance Association for the Defence of Personal Rights
may have initially been supportive of the new Act, but it soon had
misgivings. By January 1886, Lucy Wilson, the editor of the organisation's journal, seemed as worried as Josephine Butler about the
enforcement of certain of the Act's clauses, in particular the clause
dealing with 'places of vicious resort' (brothels). Elizabeth
Wolstenholme Elmy was also much perturbed, and she penned a
series of letters on this theme to the journal.

SUPPRESSION OF BROTHELS

The Criminal Law Amendment Act 1885 outlawed brothel keeping
and the procurement of women for prostitution. Under summary
proceedings brothel keepers and their agents could be sentenced
by a fine up to £20 or 3 months' imprisonment with hard labour for
the first offence, and £40 or 4 months for the second and subsequent
convictions. Prosecutions of brothels rose dramatically: in the 10
years prior to the Act, an average of 86 brothels were prosecuted in
England and Wales each year; from the year of the Act up to the
First World War the average number rose to more than 1,200
(Bristow, 1977: 154). Landlords could be held responsible under the
Act if they knowingly let houses for the purpose of prostitution.
Rising pressure on such landlords from vigilance groups led to a
wariness about letting property to 'suspect' women (such a label
would apply to most women living without men). This created a
housing problem not only for women working as prostitutes and
living in lodging-house brothels, but also for any women living

with other women, and even women living on their own, although the latter did not constitute a 'brothel'. (Self-contained flats did not come under the legal definition of a 'brothel' either, but over-cautious landlords apparently did not make – or know about – the distinction.) The situation resulted inevitably – and ironically, given the aims of the instigators of the Act – in many prostitutes being forced to resort to setting up house with pimps, or, as they were called, 'bullies', to provide a cover for their work. Pimps were only too eager to provide the 'protection'.

As brothels closed, women were being thrown out into the streets with nowhere to go. Some of these women were being subsequently sent to prison on charges of vagrancy. To Lucy Wilson this was an illustration of the argument that 'forcible interference with the voluntary vice of adult persons, when it is not without external injury to others, never had done any good, and never will'. In October she had read of 'tales of cruelty'; these were continuing and their effects were now clear. Her anger was increased by the fact that upper-class brothels – 'fashionable houses' – remained virtually untouched (Wilson, 1886).

In her letters to the journal on the theme of the prosecution of brothels, Elizabeth Wolstenholme Elmy substantiated these claims. She pointed out that brothels 'after all, are the only "homes" known to many hapless women', and 'the very first step will be that she is "taken up" by some policeman as "an idle and disorderly person"' (Wolstenholme Elmy, 1886b). In an earlier letter she had quoted French repealer Ives Guyot's sharp recognition of the double moral standard at work: 'would the men of England tolerate the inspection of their habits by the police, and the *suppression* of their houses, if police morality was dissatisfied with their conduct?' (Wolstenholme Elmy, 1886a, original emphasis).

Elmy predicted the virtual re-introduction of the Contagious Diseases Acts. She presented this forewarning to 'those old fellow-workers' who 'now sanction . . . a cruel repression'. Although it was 'painful to differ so profoundly', she felt compelled to ask them:

> Have you protested against the arbitrary *arrest and examination* of women as 'unconstitutional and unjust' [when campaigning against the CD Acts] solely because they were inspected in the name of public health? Do such things become constitutional and just because they are done in the name of public morals? . . .

I say advisably '*arrest and examination*' because ... under the Prisons Act, such examinations are perfectly possible.

(Wolstenholme Elmy, 1886b, original emphasis)

The result would be that '[i]n the name of public morality and social purity our mistaken friends will have brought us back to that cruel oppression of women which they denounced and resisted when enforced in the alleged interests of the public health' (ibid).

In contrast over the following 2 years, the NVA's *The Vigilance Record*, edited by Mrs Ormiston Chant, was full of the 'good work' being done by vigilance groups in closing brothels. Yet the NVA faced a recurrent problem, namely the prostitutes' lack of inclination 'to leave their sinful life' (*The Vigilance Record*, 15 April 1887). At a conference of 'London Societies of Vigilance Committees', the NVA Secretary, William Coote, warned that:

there was a grave danger lest Vigilance Committees should concentrate solely on the closing of bad houses. To do this alone would only drive the evil deeper down ... and it was essential that every effort should be made to draw the women who lived in ... disorderly houses into a better life.

(Coote, 1887)

Despite Coote's directive, attempts at 'rescue' work seem to have been decidedly unsuccessful as far as the inhabitants of brothels were concerned. The outcome of the NVA's closing of a 'colony' of brothels in Aldershot in 1888 was a case in point. Asked what would happen to the 400 girls and children rendered homeless by their action, Coote replied in an open court that 'he was prepared to take charge of the whole of the girls and children ... provided they were anxious to make an effort to lead an honourable and honest life'. This offer was repeated several times elsewhere, but no more than 5 or 6 girls took up the offer (*The Vigilance Record*, July 1888).

According to a later and highly critical account given by the *Personal Rights Journal*, the number was possibly even lower. The journal quoted an NVA report on its response to a query concerning the homeless girls: 'the Association bravely [!] determined to take care of them, but although 34 were taken into the local hospital, only one other was found desirous of accepting the Society's PROTECTION and leading once more a pure and honest life' (*Personal Rights Journal*). The *Personal Rights Journal* sarcastically commented:

It is difficult to say whether the *bravery* of a powerful society, cramming homeless and helpless girls into a hospital where surgical outrage ... awaits them, or the eccentricity of those who were not willing to accept such *protection*, is the more remarkable. We should like to know what became of the remainder of the 400, and also whether the one lamb 'willing' to be led to the slaughter was led by the gentle hands of the Aldershot police.

(*Personal Rights Journal*, January 1889, original emphasis)

The journal christened the NVA: 'vigilant stampers upon the feeble', and observed that these 'stampers' unfortunately included women, notably Mrs Millicent Fawcett and Mrs Ormiston Chant.

In contrast to the *Personal Rights Journal*, the *Hants and Surrey Times* declared sanctimoniously:

It is not only the reputation of the town, but also the moral well-being of our young people that is imperilled by the toleration of this flagrant vice.... Demoralization must attend the sights and sounds of vice to which we are constantly exposed in our principal streets.

(*The Vigilance Record*, July 1888)

Yet, the contradiction of which the *Hants and Surrey Times* (and possibly the NVA) seemed unaware, was that the closing of brothels was likely to increase the amount of soliciting taking place in the streets. The immediate outcome of this particular case was a definite *rise* in 'the sights and sounds of vice'. For of those prostitutes unwilling to be 'led to the slaughter', 90 marched through Aldershot in protest, 4 abreast, singing as they went. *The Vigilance Record* was shocked: 'a very bad sight was witnessed' (ibid).

THE 'EMPIRE' AND MRS LAURA ORMISTON CHANT

As editor of *The Vigilance Record*, Laura Chant actively sanctioned the removal of brothels. Her desire to close down brothels was part of a wider vision which involved the regulation and censoring of all public 'temptations to vice'. Brothels stood on the border of the worlds of the public and the private – to the uninitiated, they could 'pass' as private residences; as part of the culture of an area and a community, their presence was public knowledge. Brothels needed abolishing, not regulating, as far as Laura Chant was concerned, but other public places needed active supervision. Here the law was required to stand hand in hand with active 'protection' and 'guidance' from those in the 'know': 'what is wanted ... is the appointment of inspectors of both sexes, especially of capable women, to supervise the moral conduct of the streets and public places (Chant, 1902). She no doubt saw her own music hall inspections as a contribution to this moral supervision.

When Mrs Chant visited the 'Empire' in 1894, it was not the first time that she had 'inspected' a music hall. From June 1888 until April 1889 the NVA's monthly journal *The Vigilance Record* ran a series entitled 'Amused London', chronicling the sallying forth of Mrs Chant and a woman companion to various music halls in both the West and East Ends. What she found there may have amused London, but it certainly did not amuse Mrs Chant. The worst case was a West End Theatre of Varieties (unnamed by Mrs Chant) where the lack of clothing in the ballet and the indecent suggestiveness of other performances were 'surpassed in indecency by the conduct of the audience. The whole was nothing but an open market for vice ... the wretched painted women openly plying their horrible trade, ... the guilty, foul-eyed men, seeking whom they might devour' (Chant, 1889). The scene struck her as unearthly in its nastiness: 'It was as though we had seen with Dante the vision of ... the unhallowed victims of their own lusts, swept round and round in never-ending circles by the storming gusts of their unchained passions' (Chant, 1889).

In contrast, a well-known working-class music hall in Paddington 'was immeasurably superior, in moral tone and decency' to the 'fashionable' (read 'upper class') West End equivalent. 'Of course there was vulgarity, but vulgarity of a downright honest, homely kind, unseasoned by vicious jests or indecent allusions. Indeed the audience seemed of a fresher and more wholesome type, more child-like in nature, easily amused.' Unlike the 'educated gentlemen' of the West End, they did not require 'either vice or indecency to whet their jaded appetites' (Chant, 1888). Nevertheless, Mrs Chant held to the general principle that there was 'a necessity for stepping in to provide amusements for the people' (Chant, 1894a).

In her references to music halls she was deploying both the social purist's view of the male aristocracy as lascivious and debauched, and the philanthropist's view of the working class as 'child-like' and in need of direction. Like other members of the middle class, she also saw the working class and their leisure pursuits as a threat; like other social-purity feminists, the leisure pursuits of her own class were equally of deep concern. Music halls were predominantly working class, but the West End 'Palaces of Varieties', of which the Empire was one, attracted many upper- and middle-class men, including aristocrats, army officers, students and clerks. In relation to the working class, Mrs Chant was primarily concerned with the performances: the demoralising effects on audience and performers alike of near-nakedness, and the insidious sexual innuendo imparted to certain songs. She was certain that everyone would agree on the indecency of nakedness: 'The most advanced would draw the line at the costume of our first parents before the Fall' (Chant, 1889). In relation to the upper and middle classes, her concern was more with the behaviour of the audience, above all the presence of 'women openly plying their horrible trade'. It was the *explicitness* which appeared to most offend and alarm her – not just in the music halls of course, but also on London's streets.

WOMEN AND PUBLIC SPACES

Laura Chant's concern was partly about the danger of demoralisation, but it was surely also about the desire to transform the streets and sites of public entertainment into places where women could move freely without fear of attack or of the label of unrespectability. 'Respectable' women in this period were increasingly entering the public domain. They were there in various guises – as philanthropists, missionaries, Poor Law guardians, clerical workers, civil servants, teachers. . . . Walking around in public places was fraught with difficulties and dangers. The term 'public woman' meant the same as the term 'street walker'; both implied that the public world excluded respectable women. It was reserved for men and those women who 'immorally' serviced them. Feminists then, as now, wanted the streets and other public places to be safe for women, both literally and symbolically. For women to be unable to venture into such places without being labelled 'immoral', necessarily acted as a constraint upon their freedom of movement. Breaking down the barriers of that constraint was obviously part of the feminist agenda. As one feminist journal expressed it: ' . . . it is our business to see that in this nineteenth century there is not a street in London where a woman may not walk safely, and even not be afraid to ask her way' (*The Pioneer*, August 1887).

WOMEN'S WORK WITHIN PHILANTHROPY AND LOCAL GOVERNMENT

Earlier I suggested that women's role within philanthropy and local government played a part in the move of certain feminists towards a 'repressive' moral politics. Throughout the nineteenth century, feminists, including feminist repealers, were often engaged in philanthropic activities. By the end of the century, many of them began to move into local government (see Hollis, 1989). It was a logical move, for they saw local government as they saw philanthropy: involving the extension of women's home influence – their domesticating and 'civilizing' role – into the wider world. Women active in local government thought of themselves as engaging in municipal housekeeping. It may surprise readers today that women, excluded from central government until 1918, were able to play an important part in local government several decades earlier. From 1869, unmarried and widowed female ratepayers were able to vote in local elections, although it was not until 1907 that women were finally allowed to stand for election in borough and county councils. However, from 1870 *any* woman could stand for the new school boards, but they had to be a ratepayer to vote for them. (Thus in this case it was easier for a woman to stand as a candidate than be a voter!) Female ratepayers could vote for Poor Law boards, but for some time it was unclear whether women were eligible to serve on them. However, in 1875 one woman stood successfully for a London Poor Law union, and by 1895 there were over 800 elected women. They were encouraged by the Society for Promoting the Return of Poor Law Guardians, or Women Guardians Society, as it was known.

If women who entered local government were motivated by philanthropic sentiment, many women were additionally concerned to forward women's rights, including women's claim to political citizenship. As Hollis (1987) points out, by the mid-1880s women on school boards and Poor Law boards were helping to shape education and poor relief, but the built environment – its streets, houses, public health and policing – was still outside their remit, and in the hands of (male) town councillors. Women's concern to influence the management of public spaces stemmed partly from the desire to facilitate women's entry into a world hostile to their presence. With the 1888 Local Government Act there seemed to be an opening for women. The Act posited that 'every person shall be qualified to be elected and be a councillor who is qualified to elect to the office of a councillor' (Hollis, 1987: 306). The fact that unmarried and widowed female ratepayers were qualified to elect, prompted a number of middle-class women to form the Society for Promoting Women as County Councillors (later called the Women's Local Government Society). With their backing, Jane Cobden and Lady Sandhurst were returned as councillors in January 1889, although Lady Sandhurst was unseated 2 months later by a court action which deemed her election unconstitutional. (The court ruled that if Parliament had not expressly included women, their exclusion must be assumed (Hollis, 1987: 311).) In the meantime, if women could not be councillors themselves, a number were at least determined to pressurise male councillors as much as possible in the pursuit of certain objectives. What objectives were these?

An examination of the membership of the Women Guardians Society and the Women's Local Government Society reveals that members were involved in a network of Liberal, philanthropic, temperance and social purity organisations, including allegiance to the NVA. Mrs Ormiston Chant, for example, belonged to the Women's Liberal Federation, was a temperance campaigner and a founder member of both the Women Guardians' Society and the NVA. (Indeed, the NVA actively supported the election of female Poor Law Guardians.) Thus the objectives of women active in local government tended to relate to issues of morality, or 'social purity', to use the term of the period. The LCC was perceived as a possible vehicle for the furtherance of social purity concerns, not least in its role as the licenser of London's music halls. To ensure 'decency', Mrs Chant and other members of the NVA encouraged the newly created LCC's 'Theatre and Music Halls Committee' to 'vigilantly watch our entertainments, and vigorously repress whatever is clearly contrary to good morals' (*The Vigilance Record*, April 1889). The LCC did not need much encouragement, for until 1907 it was controlled by the 'Progressives'. Known as 'Municipal Puritans' or 'Municipal Socialists', the Progressive councillors were mainly Nonconformist, and represented 'new liberal', fabian and trade union interests. Viewing alcoholism and moral corruption as the chief causes of working-class social unrest (see Summerfield, 1981) they were as keen as any member of the NVA, indeed several of the councillors *were* members of the NVA, to rid music halls of impropriety, vice and alcohol and turn them into sites for 'wholesome' family entertainment. The Progressives institutionalised vigilance in 1890 with the introduction of an LCC inspectorate: 23 inspectors 'to devote their attention chiefly to the nature of the performance and to the character and conduct of the audience, especially the female portion thereof' (Theatre and Music Halls Committee of the LCC, 31 July 1890, quoted in Pennybacker, 1986: 127).

Given its moral politics, it was no surprise that the LCC upheld Mrs Chant's complaint at its Licensing Committee in October 1894. Further, in her role as voluntary inspector, Mrs Chant was thought to have taken action as a responsible and morally concerned citizen – precisely the kind of civic activity dear to the heart of many on the LCC. The 'Empire' was informed that its licence would only be renewed if alcoholic drink was banned from the auditorium, and the Promenade – the site of 'Empire' assignations between prostitutes and clients – was abolished.

I would suggest, from the above, that the shift in the attitudes of certain feminist repealers towards the state is partly explained by their involvement in local government. Of course feminist repealers were never a homogeneous grouping; it cannot be assumed, for example, that all members of the 1870s Ladies National Association (the feminist repeal group) were libertarians like Josephine Butler and Elizabeth Wolstenholme Elmy, even though they were united in their opposition to the CD Acts. Differences, no doubt, were there below the surface, to emerge at a later date. However, whatever particular opinions these women held about the state in the 1870s, by the 1880s and 1890s the attitudes of many were changing. With women's entry into local government, and their entry into the national government supposedly in the offing, hostility towards the phenomenon of state intervention began to wane. Included here was their attitude towards the police. They believed that if women could be an active *part* of state bodies, including the police force (indeed there were feminists arguing for women police from the late nineteenth century on (see Bland, 1985)) these bodies would be transformed accordingly. Such was the optimism of feminists of the day.

This shift in some feminists' attitudes towards the state contributes one small clue as to why certain women turned to repressive action. Another piece to the puzzle lies in the very *practice* of philanthropy which these women brought with them to their work on issues of morality. Whatever the benefits to its recipients, philanthropy clearly entailed their subjection to specific forms of surveillance, including the imposition of middle-class norms of domesticity. It is in this sense that philanthropy has been analysed as involving a 'familialist strategy' – intervention at the level of the family in order to control women's and children's sexual and social behaviour and to remake working-class culture (see Donzelot, 1979). To transform the character of a class, it was thought necessary to influence the disciplining of children, and to persuade mothers to play a key role in such disciplining. Positively, as Judith Walkowitz points out (Walkowitz, 1984), the encouragement of 'women's home influence' provided the rationale for a mother's right to control sexual access to her daughters, thereby subverting the man's authority in the home. Negatively, it promoted a custodial, if caring, relationship between mothers and daughters, relating to the middle-class Victorian idea of the sanctity of childhood (which working-class parents were frequently thought to be violating) and a view of adolescence as a period of social dependency – in contrast to the reality of most working-class (employed) adolescents' lives. To the middle classes, *all* girls needed 'protection', or rather, 'protective surveillance' – from themselves, from men, and from 'unsuitable' company. These attitudes tended to pervade the actions of those feminists involved in social purity campaigning. The desire to administer 'protective surveillance' was likely to be 'repressive' in its implications. It was crucially related to the dominant ideas about female sexuality.

FEMALE MODESTY AND SEXUALITY

Josephine Butler and Elizabeth Wolstenholme Elmy may have been horrified by their former colleagues' repressive actions, but most Butlerites and repressive moralists shared an attitude towards female sexuality that had 'protective surveillance' within its logic. Judith Walkowitz describes feminists' response to girls that they came across during their philanthropic work:

> Butlerites ... registered the same feelings of repugnance and ambivalence toward incorrigible girls as they had earlier toward unrepentant prostitutes. For them as well as for more repressive moralists, the desire to protect young girls thinly masked coercive impulses to control their voluntary sexual impulses.
>
> (Walkowitz, 1980: 249)[1]

The 'repugnance and ambivalence' stemmed from their view of women as 'pure', inherently modest, and barely sexual – unless they had the misfortune to 'fall'. To say a woman had 'fallen' implied that she had lost her modesty, and become quite 'other'. The 'fall' of a young girl was instigated by her having been 'mentally debauched by licentious novels or lewd companionships; or in some way roused to unholy passion' (Moral Reform Union, n.d.: 2). However, many repealers were aware of the vulnerability of working-class women to the vagaries of the labour market. For example, when the NVA asked for rescue workers' views on the causes of prostitution, the replies cited 'extreme poverty' as well as 'vanity, idleness and frivolity' in relation to women; for male clients, it was 'sensuality' (*The Vigilance Record*, 15 January 1888).

Despite recognising the possible contribution of financial hardship in women's resort to prostitution, feminists tended to view a woman's 'fall' as heralding her total transformation. The position of the feminist social purity organisation the Moral Reform Union was not untypical:

> Modesty and a chaste deportment are a young girl's birth right and her choicest adornment ... But when the beast and the harlot have taken the woman's place, there is no depth of shameful sensuality into which she is not prepared to sink.
>
> (Moral Reform Union n.d. : 2)

However, before 'the beast and harlot' had 'taken the woman's place', the prostitute who was a *victim* of circumstances could still be saved – whether the circumstances be economic hardship or male 'seduction'. She could never of course be *fully* saved, for 'purity and innocence once lost we know but too well can never be regained' (*Woman's Signal*, 1 November 1894). According to Dr

Elizabeth Blackwell, another active feminist member of the NVA, prostitutes, if not caught in time, became 'demons', 'human tigers who delight in destruction and torture' (Blackwell, 1887: 35). She had clear ideas on the need to distinguish between the woman who remained a prostitute and the woman who was prepared to change. She offered this advice:

> The tenderest compassion may be shown to the poor creature who *ceases* to be a prostitute; ... but do nothing to raise the condition of prostitutes as such, any more than you would try to improve the condition of murderers and thieves.
>
> (Blackwell, 1881: 17, original emphasis)

The distinction between the reclaimable and the unreclaimable prostitute was akin to philanthropy's distinction between the deserving and the undeserving poor.

Such ideas informed Laura Chant's view of the performers and prostitutes at the 'Empire'. In relation to the performers, she was sure that 'the unhappy girls in the ballet and choruses ... had lost something if they did not feel the loss of clothing' (Chant, 1894). She was implying, of course, that they had lost their modesty and sense of shame. She was also implying that if they were 'rescued' in time, they might still be saved. Her greatest condemnation of fallen womanhood she reserved for the 'Empire' prostitutes. She was insistent that there was a clear distinction to be made between women such as these, who were engaged in 'guilded vice', and poor women who worked the street. While she saw the former as having calculatingly chosen their profession, she viewed the latter as *victims*. When accused of forcing the 'Empire' prostitutes back out on to the streets and thus *adding* to street prostitution, she defended herself by claiming that these women were not off the streets in the first place, since the 'Empire' explicitly stated that street walkers were refused entry. She referred to the 'Empire' prostitutes as those 'who minister entirely to the demands of lust, and who love darkness and secrecy because their lives are evil' (Chant, 1894). They sounded like Dr Blackwell's 'demons'. As for the street walker, Laura Chant was at pains to emphasise that her house had 'always been open as a refuge to the poor creatures' (Chant, 1894). Although innocence could never of course be regained, some street walkers were reclaimable. The 'Empire' women were beyond the pale. This justified her belief that ' ... the stern aid of the magistrate must be invoked against the persistent transgressor, the hand of Christian charity must be the remedy to help not yet hardened and repentant ones' (Chant, 1902: 134).

VICTIMS OF VICE AND THEIR LIBERTY

The Personal Rights Association, highly critical of the NVA's repressive actions, objected especially to its attack not on the instigators of 'criminal vice', but on the 'helpless victims': 'the *repression* of immorality by crushing its helpless victims ... is ... miscalled morality [but] represents nothing better than outward indecency' (*Personal Rights Journal*, January 1889, original emphasis). Josephine Butler made a similar criticism – the NVA's work entailed:

> a constant tendency towards *external* pressure, and inside that a tendency to let the pressure fall almost exclusively on women, because it is difficult, they say, to get at men. It is dangerous work, in reference to personal liberty, but few people care for liberty or personal rights now.
>
> (Butler, 1896, personal letter, original emphasis)

In contrast, the NVA and the feminists active within it, such as Laura Chant, Millicent Fawcett and Elizabeth Blackwell, thought of their vigilance work as neither harmful to immorality's victims, nor as a curtailment of liberty. On the contrary, they assumed that the removal of 'vice' and the alternatives which they presented, *helped* the victims. They believed their actions offered the hand of reclamation to reclaimable prostitutes, and gave freedom from immorality to that other group of 'victims of vice', namely 'ordinary citizens', including respectable women like themselves, who wished to be able to enter public spaces without fear of immoral sights and dangers. In relation to the idea of 'liberty', Millicent Fawcett turned the issue on its head: 'Some ... appear to think that any curtailment of the liberty of vice is an unjustifiable curtailment of the liberty of the subject. ... I think that freedom in vice is an unjustifiable curtailment of the liberty of the subject' (Fawcett, 1893). To Laura Chant:

> A great deal of well-meant nonsense is talked about the 'liberty of the subject', whenever there is ... effort to clear the streets. Some good people seem to be so zealous in defending the vicious from injustice that it seems as if they were in danger of

forgetting that vice is in itself a colossal injustice, an infringement of the liberty of the subject.

(Chant, 1902: 129)

While the liberty of the 'ordinary citizen' was at risk in the face of the unregenerate prostitute and other agents of vice, the regenerate prostitute needed *her* 'liberty' *rescued from* a life of vice. 'Saving' the prostitute was seen as the restoration of her liberty.

The NVA's activities did not always have the desired outcome, as we have seen. Their actions in closing brothels largely resulted not in the reclamation of prostitutes, but in the prostitutes' homelessness and increased harassment on the streets. However, rather than seeing this as a failed project, the repressive purity feminists interpreted it as an example of the hardened, unreclaimable nature of the prostitutes concerned, illustrated, for example, by the 'very bad sight' in Aldershot of women marching in protest. In the case of the prostitutes at the 'Empire', repressive purity feminists did not think of them as victims either, but as women who had calculatingly chosen a life of 'vice', and whose livelihoods deserved to be destroyed.

The repressive purity feminists shared with their less repressive sisters the desire to bring about a transformation in public and private morality, especially in the sexual relations between men and women. They appeared to believe that one of the best means to this end, at this point in time, lay with the 'domestication' and 'civilising' of the public world through philanthropic and statist interventions. Their wish to transform the public world for the benefit of all, and especially for respectable women like themselves, was part of a wider feminist vision in which women had freedom of movement in all spheres of society. Part of their work involved addressing issues of sexual violence, providing support to victims of male assault and campaigning for changes in unjust laws. Their views on female sexuality, however, and their concomitant distinction between repentant and unrepentant prostitutes, or victims and calculating 'demons', engendered 'protective surveillance' in their approach to prostitution. Coupled with their optimistic belief that their own presence within state bodies would radically change the nature of these bodies, repressive purity feminists acted in and through the state in an effort to transform the sexual morality of the time.

These women cannot be dismissed as simply 'prying prudes' or 'interfering busybodies, however undesirable the means to their feminist ends may seem to us today. It is worth recognising that in our approach to current issues of pornography, prostitution and the sex industry, many of the same dilemmas and difficulties remain as to how to use the law and how to take issue with beliefs and practices which we, as feminists, find unacceptable. As in the past, there is no one feminist position, and there is no one feminist answer to these problems.

ACKNOWLEDGEMENTS

Thanks to Judy Greenway, Dave Phillips and Martin Durham for their many helpful comments, and to Carol Smart for her patience in waiting for this chapter's completion.

NOTES

1 See Wood (1982) and Walkowitz (1984).

Chapter 3

Child sexual abuse and the regulation of women
Variations on a theme

Carol-Ann Hooper

The current wave of recognition of child sexual abuse is not the first in the history of child-protection work. From the 1870s for roughly 60 years, intermittent anxieties emerged and attempts at legal reform were made, culminating in a specific campaign on sexual offences against children initiated by feminists in the 1930s. At the end of this period, however, the criminal justice system was still hopelessly ineffective, the campaign fizzled out, and a public silence ensued (broken briefly during the 1950s) until the 1970s, when feminists again brought the issue to public attention. In both the earlier period and the present one, a number of interest groups have promoted and laid claims to the issue, offering competing definitions. Feminist definitions locating the problem in the social construction of masculinity have commonly been marginalised from the policy agenda.

Child sexual abuse is itself a site of informal social control by men over women. As girls who are victimised themselves, as partners of abusive men and as mothers and primary carers of sexually abused children, the sexual abuse of children operates to restrict women's autonomy and control of their own lives. The responses of voluntary and statutory agencies to child sexual abuse have also been centrally concerned with the regulation of women, much more so than with the control of men who abuse. In the earlier period, it was the behaviour of sexually abused girls themselves that was most subject to surveillance, although often in the name of their future as mothers. Today, it is the mothers of sexually abused children whose behaviour is the prime concern of child protection agencies.

The shift from girls to their mothers is attributable to two main trends. First, increased attention through the present century first to children's physical needs and later to their psychological needs, within an ideological context which defines child welfare as women's private business, has generated redefinitions of motherhood which accord women increased responsibilities. Definitions of fatherhood have been much less implicated (if at all) by attention to child welfare, despite the evidence now available that men far outnumber women as sexual abusers of children and play a more or less equal role in physical abuse (Stark and Flitcraft, 1988; Gordon, 1989). Second, state intervention in the home to protect children has gained greater (although by no means uncontested) acceptability. The voluntary activities of philanthropists and charitable organisations in the late-nineteenth century, to which contemporary child protection work owes its roots (Behlmer, 1982; Ferguson, 1990), have been replaced by a child-abuse management system which attempts to co-ordinate the activities of a wide range of professionals and statutory agencies. The combined effect of these trends has been to legitimate greater surveillance of mothers, alongside a still-limited commitment of resources to public services to contribute to the work and costs of childcare.

This chapter considers both periods of anxiety about child sexual abuse to illustrate the variety of ways in which women have been constructed in regulatory discourses. In the first period, I focus on how the construction of the problem changed, influenced by changing social anxieties and the strengths and orientations of social movements. In the later period, I discuss the alternative constructions of motherhood involved in contemporary discourses on child sexual abuse, and their influence on and resistance by mothers and social workers, the prime actors in the protection of children. In this section I draw on my contemporary study of mothers of sexually abused children, which involved interviews with both mothers and social workers (Hooper, 1990).

The analysis of both periods is necessarily selective and the focus on girls in the early period and their mothers in the contemporary period to some extent schematic. The greater emphasis on protecting children today is certainly not unproblematic for girls who are sexually abused, and the control of their sexuality is clearly still an issue in medical, child protection and judicial discourse (see Mitra, 1987; Kitzinger, 1988). Moreover, from its nineteenth-century beginnings, child protection work in England has sought where possible to enforce rather than replace parental responsibility for children and in doing so has reflected and perpetuated gendered definitions of proper parenting (Ferguson, 1990). In child-protection practice, there has probably therefore been as much continuity as change. However, constructions of women are continually renegotiated in specific contexts and this chapter seeks to identify some sources of variability.

There has been some speculation recently that the current anxiety about child sexual abuse is not simply a product of changed social anxieties and political movements, but a response to a new and growing problem (see O'Hagan, 1989; Gledhill and others, 1989). Before discussing the historical shifts in visibility and definitions therefore, it is worth reviewing briefly the available evidence on incidence.

ON THE INCIDENCE OF CHILD SEXUAL ABUSE

It is difficult to unearth the history of a problem kept so invisible. The most reliable sources of evidence on historical trends are contemporary surveys of adults using age-stratified samples. These are limited in scope by the lifespan and age of those interviewed, and by problems of memory, but the evidence of two such surveys, both conducted in the USA, is instructive. Russell (1984) found that incestuous abuse, but not extrafamilial child sexual abuse, had increased over the years 1916 to 1961, although the peak occurred in 1956. It is possible however that memories of incestuous abuse were more deeply buried for older women, for whom the subject had been unspeakable for so much of their lives. Finkelhor *et al.*'s (1990) more recent survey found no consistent upward trend over time. Lower rates of abuse were reported by women aged over 60 but those born 1955–67 reported no higher level of abuse than their immediate predecessors.

Both studies, however, suggest that the most significant fluctuations have coincided with war. Women born during the Second World War reported the highest levels of abuse in both surveys. Russell's analysis of period rates found that the incidence of incestuous abuse declined during both world wars, and increased immediately after. Extrafamilial child sexual abuse also declined during the Second World War and increased after, although in contrast it increased during the First World War. Although other fluctuations cannot be linked to war, these findings are illustrative of one of the many dilemmas child sexual abuse raises. Children tend to be safest from sexual abuse in the absence of men, but it is in part men's separation from children which makes them a threat when they return.

Since it is some years since any of those interviewed were children, these studies do not answer the question of whether child sexual abuse is currently increasing. It is highly likely, however, that the rapid increase during the 1980s in the number of cases of child sexual abuse on child protection registers[1] held by local authorities reflects increased reporting by members of the public, increased awareness and detection by professionals and/or increased use of the child protection register in the management of cases.

Nor do these studies reach back into the nineteenth century. Gordon's (1989) study of child protection records in Boston between 1880–1960, however, found a consistent level of 10% of cases involving incest throughout the period, despite fluctuating levels of public awareness.

It seems safe to assume that whatever its exact incidence child sexual abuse is not a new problem. This should not be surprising, since the social conditions which support it have remained consistent – the construction of masculine sexuality as predatory and not requiring reciprocity, the eroticisation of dominance, and the lack of responsibility men have for childcare.

It is not in fact correct to say that child sexual abuse has been wholly invisible. Rather, it has at certain periods been partially visible, its definition as a problem mediated through other social anxieties about 'the family', sexuality and reproduction. It is often these other concerns – with the 'health of the race' in the 1900s, or with the 'decline of the traditional family' in the 1980s, for example – that have shaped the dominant discourses.

1870s to 1930s: FROM VICTIMS TO DELINQUENTS AND LAW TO MEDICINE

Public awareness of what we would now call child sexual abuse arose in the 1870s in the context of concern about child prostitution. Shortly after, the National Society for the Prevention of Cruelty to Children (NSPCC), formed by philanthropic reformers in 1889, drew attention also to sexual abuse in the home. Up until the end of the First World War, it referred regularly (if euphemistically) to these in its annual reports, indicating that they were far more common than would easily be believed.[2] Other nineteenth-century reformers, too, encountered incestuous abuse, most notably during the investigation of housing conditions (Wohl, 1978). Campaigns were waged by the social purity movement (primarily the National Vigilance Association (NVA)), by the NSPCC itself and by feminist groups, focusing initially on legal reforms to facilitate an effective response from the criminal justice system both to incestuous and extrafamilial abuse.

Some successes were achieved in these, and two major pieces of legislation concerning sexual assault were passed during this period. Neither was unproblematic. The Criminal Law Amendment Act 1885, which raised the age of consent for sexual intercourse from 13 to 16, was supported by a range of groups brought together in a short-lived coalition. This Act could be and was used to prosecute men, including fathers, for sexual abuse. However, by portraying young prostitutes as sexually innocent, passive victims of individual evil men, the reformers had also paved the way for the increased surveillance of working-class girls and diverted attention from the economic reasons why many engaged in prostitution (Gorham, 1978). The potential for 'protection' to become control of female sexuality is a recurring theme in responses to child sexual abuse. The Punishment of Incest Act 1908, again supported by a range of groups, made incest a criminal, as opposed to an ecclesiastical offence, for the first time (Bailey and Blackburn, 1979). Calls for legislation specific to incest had been made from the 1890s, suggesting the inclusion of assaults by men in positions of authority, including employers, schoolmasters and guardians under this label (*The Vigilance Record*, December 1895). The Act passed excluded even stepfathers, adopting consanguinity as the defining feature, after debates which were concerned far more with the regulation of sexuality than the protection of children. Further campaigns achieved amendments to the 1885 Act, including the raising of the age of consent for indecent assault from 13 to 16 (1922), the partial removal of 'the defence of reasonable belief' (that the man had believed a girl was over the age of consent when she was not) (1922) and extending the time limit under which prosecutions could be brought, from 3 months (1885), to 6 months (1904), 9 months (1922) and finally to 12 months in 1928.

However, when a government review was conducted in 1925, a number of further problems were noted with the law and its administration. The Report of the Departmental Committee on Sexual Offences against Young Persons (1925) noted that many cases were unreported, that many more, once reported, were sifted out before reaching court for lack of proof, and that for those that did reach court, the acquittal rate was unusually high. Its recommendations involved measures to ease the strain of the process on children (including the greater use of women as police, doctors and magistrates in such cases, and the quicker and less formal conducting of court proceedings) and changes to the rules of evidence (since in effect a higher level of proof was required for sexual offences than in most others, making convictions almost impossible). A recommendation was also made that the age of consent be raised to 17, although four members of the Committee dissented, three wanting no change and one wanting it raised to 18.

The report did not concern itself only with the criminal law. It made a range of recommendations on prevention, and also on changes to the civil law to facilitate the removal of children from their homes. However, it was the role of the criminal law that was the spark for action, since groups hoping to see these recommendations incorporated in the forthcoming Children's Bill were disappointed when it was published in 1932.[3] Resolutions were passed at various organisations' annual conferences, and the feminist Association of Moral and Social Hygiene, then led by Alison Neilans, a former active suffragist, held a small specific conference in November 1932. From this a Joint Committee on Sexual Offences against Children was established, representing 14 national organisations (including AMSH itself, the NVA, the National Council of Women, the British Social Hygiene Council, the National Council of Mental Hygiene and the Howard League for Penal Reform, amongst others). Representatives of these groups met over the next 3 years, with the aim of agreeing a limited bill with a good chance of success around which to mobilise a campaign. They were not able to do so. They dissolved in 1935 having published a brief report and two leaflets[4] and little further campaigning occurred on the problem of child sexual abuse.

I am not suggesting that had they achieved further legal reforms, this would have solved the problem of child sexual abuse. The law was and is one of the ways in which patriarchal power is maintained and has rarely provided protection for women or girls from male violence, as feminists have frequently pointed out.

Furthermore, many of the recommendations of the 1925 report, on which the campaign focused, did not require legislation. It is probably more important that the degree of disagreement within the campaigns, in which the significance of the criminal law was a key issue, weakened the commitment to any further action. The result, however, was that the major legislation passed in the wake of the government review, the Children and Young Persons Act 1933, focused on the control of juvenile delinquency (defined for girls in relation to their sexuality) and on the removal of children 'in moral danger' or 'beyond parental control' from their parents (identifying parental, primarily maternal, neglect as the problem). How did this reconstruction of the problem come about? And how, then, did the issue disappear from public attention effectively until the 1970s? Viewing the period of 60 years or so very broadly, two major shifts seem significant. First, social anxieties about the 'health of the race' from the turn of the century resulted in an increasing significance attached to motherhood in the latter part of the period. Changing concepts of childhood and adolescence at the same time made the problem of defining abuse, represented by debates on the age of consent, increasingly contentious. Second, popular support for the social purity movement whose main focus had been legal reform had declined, the strength of the medical profession which offered a new alliance of science and morality in the discourse of social hygiene had increased, and the declining feminist movement increasingly sided with the latter rather than the former. The disputes that occurred in debates on child sexual abuse during the 1930s reflected these broader changes.

The growing influence of Freudian ideas in the inter-war years no doubt also played its part. Freud's volte-face which led him to attribute his women patients' accounts of sexual abuse to incestuous fantasy has been well documented elsewhere (Rush, 1984; Masson, 1985). But the reluctance to believe children's accounts, which was displayed by some (though not all) members of the Joint Committee, and to name the abuse of paternal power, was neither new, nor is it passed today.

The health of the race and the rise of maternalism

Around the turn of the century, the health of the population became a major national concern. Anxieties about the falling birth rate, high infant mortality, the poverty uncovered by Booth and Rowntree and the poor physical conditions of recruits to the Boer War combined in a rising fear that the nation's health was degenerating. This fear continued and increased during the war as deaths at the front increased, and the birth rate continued to fall. In response, childhood, motherhood and sex were all accorded new meanings. Child protection and child welfare reforms were facilitated by these concerns, since children were the raw material to be safeguarded in the name of national efficiency. Motherhood became defined as crucial to child health. High infant mortality and physical deterioration were attributed not to poverty but to ignorant motherhood, the solution seen as the education of working-class mothers better to fulfil their national duty as 'guardians of the race' (Davin, 1978; Bland, 1982). Sex became the key to the question of population, both in its effects on the health of the individual (particularly via VD), and on the future of the population (via the association of VD with sterility, and the higher infant mortality of unmarried mothers) (Weeks, 1989). At the same time, the notion of adolescence as a distinct period of development, and one of particular significance for the channelling of sexuality towards responsible parenthood, emerged.

These shifts influenced the way sexual abuse was constructed in a number of ways. First, concern focused often not on the victimised girl herself but on her potential offspring as the true victim. In the Commons debate on the Incest Bill 1908, the main argument put forward by Mr Herbert Samuel, Home Office Under-Secretary, for criminalising incest was that 'it might entail consequences of a disastrous kind on the offspring which sometimes followed from such intercourse, and from that point of view society had a special interest that should lead to steps being taken to put a stop to it' (Hansard, 26 June 1908, col. 284).

Second, and linked to this, the response to the victimised girl increasingly reflected concerns about her potential performance as a mother. The Royal Commission on the Care and Control of the Feeble-Minded which sat in 1908 heard evidence that 'feeble-minded' girls were particularly vulnerable to sexual assault, that many had illegitimate children as a result, and that such children were likely to be 'imbeciles, or degenerates, or criminals'. Its response was to recommend the segregation of such girls in order to prevent them from reproducing themselves.[5]

The NVA, whose aim was to transform sexual behaviour towards a high standard of chastity in both men and women, increasingly adopted the new concern for the national stock in place of the moral language of vice and corruption it had previously used. Germany was criticised for allowing earlier marriage in order to counter the falling birth rate, since to 'prematurely exploit young girlhood' would not pay off 'from the racial point of view' (*The Vigilance Record*, October 1915: 79–80). In 1922 an article in the *Evening Standard* was cited approvingly, arguing against the use of the 'reasonable cause to believe' defence as follows:

> (the law) should, in fact, regard adolescent women as at least as important as adolescent fish or breeding animals. It is an offence to shoot game in the close season, or to take fish below a certain size, and no 'reasonable cause' can be pleaded. Why should there be a necessity for a big loophole regarding the age of consent?
>
> (*The Vigilance Record*, September 1922: 59)

Motherhood and promiscuity were constructed as separate routes by the social hygiene movement during this period, and the concern of the newly developing sex education was primarily to divert girls from 'promiscuity' towards responsible and healthy motherhood (Bland, 1982). Hence this concern with motherhood facilitated the shift of concern from abuse itself to its consequences (perceived through the lens of women as reproducers), since the diversion of girls from 'promiscuity', from the risk of VD and from unmarried motherhood (all of which were for some girls the consequence of sexual abuse) became a high priority. It was considerably easier and less threatening to prevailing power structures to patrol and control girls in all these circumstances, sending them to homes for their reform, than effectively to counter the abuses of men in the home or on the street.

This concern to preserve girls for their future reproductive roles was one continued justification for those who sought the further raising of the age of consent. Debates on this issue were complex, however, and are not adequately represented as concerned solely with the repressive regulation of female sexuality sought by social purity or a feminist obsession with male vice. Feminists in the 1885 debates were sometimes drawn into an alliance with social purity in opposition to the attempts of upper-class men to preserve their unfettered access to working-class girls, losing sight temporarily of the risks of such legislation for the civil liberties of young women (Gorham, 1978). Despite increasing recognition of the problems the age of consent brought, however, many continued to be ambivalent. While purity campaigners sought the protection of girls 'from themselves', some feminists noted more their protection from exposure to the full rigours of the double standard (e.g. *The Vote*, 11 May 1912). The age of consent marked the dividing line around which the contradictions of women's responsibility for sexuality, both less and more responsible than men, polarised (Bland, 1982). Below it girls were perceived as without responsibility, justifying (sometimes oppressive) protection. But above it, they bore responsibility not only for themselves but also for men, as illustrated by the prosecution of women for soliciting.

Later, the arguments of some feminists for raising the age of consent to 18 were allied to the cause of sexual equality by calling for the raising of the age of criminal responsibility also to 18. This was justified by the new medicalised concept of adolescence as an inherently unstable time when neither boys nor girls were fit to decide for themselves.[6] The NVA had by the 1930s also bowed to the new definition of adolescence although they took a different, and in this instance less repressive, approach laying strong emphasis on distinguishing between assaults on young children, and what they referred to as 'technical assaults' or 'boy and girl cases' involving 'foolish youths and precocious girls'. The 1925 report was criticised for conflating the two quite different issues and the NVA consistently attempted to exclude the latter from campaigns. Divisions on this issue continued to emerge in the 1930s, although the Joint Committee agreed from the beginning to exclude the age of consent from their remit as too contentious. The Home Office had already indicated that further legislation on the issue would get nowhere.

The third way in which concerns with motherhood influenced the construction of sexual abuse was by the new responsibilities and powers accorded women as mothers. Concern with child health and the role of mothers in securing it brought a shift towards greater emphasis on women as mothers and a lesser emphasis on women as wives. The extended length of childhood further exaggerated the role of women as mothers. As women were accorded greater powers to influence their children, attention to their own victimisation declined. Feminist groups continued in the suffrage campaigns to draw attention to the victimisation of women as well as children,[7] and to the inequity of the responsibilities accorded mothers for children when they had few legal rights and limited access to resources. But while the link between delinquency and parental neglect was not new,[8] it was firmly established in the 1933 Act. Family breakdown and working mothers became the key culprits, both seen as the result of economic deprivation (League of Nations, 1934). Many feminists by then felt the new responsibilities of motherhood offered potential for enhancing women's status in the home and pursued welfare reforms with this aim, simultaneously moving away from the earlier critique of sexual exploitation by men. Thus AMSH cited approvingly a reference to the causes of delinquency which commented 'a home without a mother is only half a home' (*The Shield*, November 1934), and in the debates on child sexual abuse of the 1930s, a National Council of Women conference observed that 'a great many problem cases would never have arisen if children had been brought up in the right knowledge' (*Scotsman*, 21 November 1933). Parent education was advocated as a preventive measure, as was the speeding up of slum clearance. The former in effect accorded mothers the responsibility for preventing sexual abuse. The latter implied that incestuous abuse was the product of overcrowded housing and did nothing to tackle the power of men within households.

Social purity, social hygiene and feminism

The weakening of the feminist critique of masculinity reflects another important shift, the relative decline of the social purity movement and the rise of social hygiene, alongside changing attitudes amongst feminists both to sex and to the law. During the late-nineteenth century, the social purity movement had mobilised a major campaign for moral reform and the suppression of vice. Their stress on criminal legislation as a means of achieving this reflected a then new perception of the state's capacity to transform sexual and moral behaviour (Mort, 1987). The NVA, for example, claimed that in Ireland where incest was a criminal offence, it did not occur (*The Vigilance Record*, December 1895). In the suffrage campaigns many feminists shared this faith in the potential role of law, despite its current male bias. The Women's Freedom League made similarly wild claims for a legal system open to the beneficial influence of women (see e.g. *The Vote*, 9 March 1912). Many (although not all) feminists had also shared social purity concerns with male lust and the double standard, campaigning for women's right to say no to unwanted sex.[9] However, by the 1930s popular support for social purity, with its explicitly moral language of sin, vice and degeneracy and adherence to criminal law as a deterrent had declined. The social hygiene movement on the other hand, which had emerged in the 1900s offering new scientific knowledges to the population debates, was well established, speaking an apparently more progressive language. Many of the same moral judgements were in fact reworked into the medical discourse of science, but social hygiene promoted a more positive image of sex with an emphasis on education and prevention as regulatory practices rather than suppression and punishment.

Many feminists by this time had moved to some degree away both from their earlier suspicion of the medical profession (derived from the involvement of the latter in the regulation of prostitution in the nineteenth century), and their faith in the efficacy of legal reform, recognising that the latter often resulted in greater surveillance of women. Increasingly, they also focused on women's right to sexual pleasure rather than on protection from sexual exploitation (Bland, 1983). Hence, they allied themselves with the seemingly more progressive forces of social hygiene. Alison Neilans was an enthusiastic representative of this trend, calling for legislation on sexual assault that would 'take people out of the category of criminals and put them into the category of mental invalids' (*Scotsman*, 21 November 1933). AMSH, in its calls for new legislation, focused entirely on the medical examination and treatment of offenders against children under 13. The medicalisation of sexual offences against young children that took place in this period was part of a broader trend occurring, although not without conflict, towards psychological explanations for crime and delinquency (Weeks, 1989). Its basis in moral criteria is illustrated by the label adopted of 'moral perversion' and by the claim made for the role of the medical profession by Dr W.D. Fairbairn: 'I submit that, since a child does not constitute a natural object of overt sexual behaviour on the part of an adult, such behaviour in itself constitutes a perverse act' (Fairbairn, 1935: 15). Such elaborate claims for a disease model were not apparently inhibited by the fact that neither the cause nor the cure had yet been found.

Neither earlier feminists nor social-purity campaigners had been hesitant in naming the construction of normal male sexuality as a problem. The medical profession, however, relied on the concept of abnormality for its claims both to seek and to treat pathology, and feminists who dissented from this were increasingly marginalised. The receptiveness of feminists to the medical model was increased both by sympathy for men's suffering in the war, and increasing interest in the problem of persistent offenders, since the case was made that treating one offender successfully would prevent a series of further assaults. Broader ideas of prevention were drawn from social hygiene's image of sex as a healthy instinct in need of channelling towards socially approved goals. The 1925 report recommended sex education and the provision of facilities for healthy indoor and outdoor recreation as preventive measures, and in some later debates allowing earlier marriage was suggested. Feminist proposals for prevention also included sex education, along with talks to parents and improved housing.

Representatives of the medical profession claimed their analysis did not affect the issue of criminal responsibility. Purity campaigners, however, saw it as a direct challenge to their ideas, and one not to be taken lying down. While some members of the NVA shifted towards a medical discourse and officially it endorsed calls for medical examination and treatment, internally members were divided, and Frederick Sempkins, the current Secretary, waged a personal campaign against 'throwing (the issue) over to the alienists'. Medical treatment was to him both a soft option, and of limited relevance, since it mattered little what was done with convicted offenders when the main problem was the impossibility of gaining convictions in the first place. The latter point (still pertinent today) seems to have fallen on deaf ears, in part because feminists (and others) were preoccupied with resisting his punitive emphasis on the law as a deterrent and occasional advocacy of flogging, in part because of the intransigence of the legal profession when faced with any proposal which addressed the problem.

While the general public had received the 1925 report well (with the exception of the proposal to raise the age of consent to 17), the legal profession had not. They objected strongly and consistently to proposals for changes in legal procedure. The report was attacked for being 'founded on the popular misconception that every prosecution is necessarily well-founded and every defence inevitably a speculative subterfuge' (*Law Journal*, 6 March 1926: 215). The recommendation for the greater involvement of women police and doctors in sexual offences received almost equal hostility, on the grounds that this would bias the system further against men. This latter argument resonates ironically with the arguments of the suffrage campaign. The Women's Freedom League for instance had claimed 'it would be quite as intelligible to expect a Tory to legislate to a Liberal's satisfaction as to expect one sex to legislate fairly for another' (*The Vote*, 19 March 1910). Given the shared assumption of inevitable difference, and 'sex antipathy' (*Law Journal*, 6 March 1926: 215), clearly the legal profession preferred the option of unfettered male bias. It was not uncommon for the intimidating nature of a court appearance for young girls to be deliberately increased by the exclusion of women magistrates and jury members from sexual assault cases (Report of the Departmental Committee on Sexual Offences against Young Persons, 1925). While in the 1930s, Sempkins located one sympathetic judge, Judge Cecil Whiteley, willing to argue for changes in procedure including relaxation of corroboration rules, and a tribunal system of questioning,[10] even he appeared to give up on so controversial a subject, and the legal advisers to the Joint Committee dismissed proposals for any change to legal procedure out of hand.

The Joint Committee dissolved in 1935, having failed to resolve the conflicts between medical and legal definitions of child sexual abuse which were frequent during the 1920s and 1930s. Both the declining strength of feminism, and the shifts in its orientation, towards a focus on sexual pleasure more than danger, on economic rather than sexual exploitation, on education rather than legal reform and on strengthening women's maternal role, all contributed further to the loss of child sexual abuse as a public issue as the medical profession took it over in its claims to a new scientific discourse on sex.

THE 1970s ON: WOMEN AS CAUSE, PROTECTION AND CONTROL

There can be few people who are not aware of the rediscovery of child sexual abuse in the present. Initiated by feminist campaigns against male violence in the 1970s, child sexual abuse became a high-profile public issue during the late 1980s and remains one today. Contemporary social anxieties about sex and the family have influenced this, and child sexual abuse has been attributed both to the 'sexual permissiveness' of the 1960s (O'Hagan, 1989), and to the 'decline of the traditional family' (Gledhill and others, 1989). Concerns about demographic changes, the increased divorce rate and proportion of lone-parent families, underly anxiety that the extent of child sexual abuse revealed by research will lead to a further escalation in 'fragmented (i.e. fatherless) families' (Fawcett, 1989). At the same time, the relative rights and powers of children, parents and the different agencies and professional groups involved in child protection, to define what constitutes abuse, remain hotly contested. The ineffectiveness of the criminal justice system has continued, despite some changes facilitated by the existence of new technology as well as a considerably stronger child protection lobby.[11] The context of response by other agencies, however, has changed.

The medical profession's dominance over the fields of both child abuse and sexuality is now well established, reflected in policy debates if not necessarily in practice. Post-war developments in child care have attributed changed significance to family life, reflected in the acquisition of new duties by local authorities, first to return children from care to their families where possible (the Children Act 1948) and then to prevent their reception into care by helping families with children at home (the Children and Young Persons Act 1963). The idealised view of family life underlying these changes retracted a little after the battering to death of Maria Colwell by her stepfather in 1973 (after being returned home to her natural mother), and the Children Act 1975 made it easier to extricate children from their natural parents.[12] Further changes are enshrined in the Children Act 1989, to be implemented in 1991, which was influenced by a series of inquiries held during the 1980s, first involving three children who died at home at the hands of their fathers or stepfathers, for whom professionals were blamed for doing too little too late,[13] and later involving 121 children suspected of being sexually abused in Cleveland, for whom professionals were accused of doing too much too soon.[14] The Act attempts again to rework the balancing act, both increasing the grounds for state intervention to protect children and setting out a new framework for partnership with parents geared to the preservation and support of parental responsibilities. Despite these shifts, childcare work throughout has focused primarily on mothers, with child abuse defined as a problem of poor mothering but separation from mothers also defined as a key traumatic event to be avoided for children. Child sexual abuse as a problem for statutory agencies landed in this context. Consequently, the surveillance of girls in the previous period has been to some extent replaced (and certainly supplemented) by the increased surveillance of women as mothers of sexually abused children.

Feminist criticisms of mother-blaming in relation to child sexual abuse have focused primarily on 'family dysfunction theory', a medical discourse preoccupied with causality, which, having shifted its focus from the individual to the family as unit, sought it in any deviation from androcentrically defined and historically specific norms (see e.g. Nelson, 1987; MacLeod and Saraga, 1988). In the dominant versions of this, sexuality as the core feature of marriage and a construction of motherhood defined in relation to children's psychological and emotional needs (both developments of the post-war period) were enshrined, as was a functionalist model of the family which defined the sexual division of labour as natural. The result was the implication of women in the cause of abuse, via sexual estrangement from their partners, the unmet needs of their children, and/or their absence from the home (e.g. CIBA Foundation, 1984), a model which has been roundly condemned by feminists, to some effect. However, the influence this model exerted over the social practices of agencies involved in child protection was never obvious, since social workers generally pay more attention to pragmatic concerns than theoretical explanations (Corby, 1987) and their resources for therapeutic work are limited. In this section I want to consider first, what influence this discourse has had on social workers (the prime actors in the surveillance of women), and on mothers themselves (the prime actors in child protection), and second, to discuss the problems and potential of the child protection discourse which I would argue is more central for both groups. Finally, I discuss the construction of motherhood in contemporary judicial discourse. While there is overlap between the constructions of women in different discourses, there are also significant differences.

Social workers, mothers and medical discourse

Social workers draw on the available professional discourses alongside other sources of knowledge, from the wider community and their own experience, in their efforts to make sense of their work (Pithouse, 1987). In my study, labels such as 'a collusive wife', and 'a dysfunctional family' were employed with little meaning in themselves as part of the process of distancing the worker from the client. Judgements such as 'she knew' or 'she disbelieved' were also made in relation to mothers of sexually abused children, despite evidence of far more complex processes involving doubt, uncertainty and ambivalence, as shorthand for 'not doing enough'. 'Enough' however was often defined with the benefit of hindsight, and the label served the purpose primarily of attributing fault (Hooper, 1990).

For social workers, 'blaming' clients, by constructing them as a 'particular sort of person' to whom it could be expected that awful things would happen is one of the main ways in which they manage 'occupational impotence' (Pithouse, 1987). Where child sexual abuse is concerned the sources of occupational impotence are numerous: the tightrope social workers must walk between criticism for unwarranted intervention in the family on the one hand and failure to protect children on the other, difficulties of gaining direct access to children and to evidence of abuse, uncertainty about both the definition of abuse and often about the best solution, an inadequate knowledge base to predict accurately the risk to children that leaving them in the care of a particular adult involves, the relatively low status of social workers in the professional networks involved in child protection compared with the medical profession and police, the inadequacy of the criminal justice system, the lack of resources both for alternative accommodation for children and therapeutic work with individuals and families, and the reluctance of some individuals and families to participate in what services are offered.

The result is high levels of anxiety. As one social worker in my study put it, 'My protectiveness to her is like an Aertex vest . . . total protection is a myth'. Since mothers are the main alternative sources of child protection, it is they who bear the brunt of social workers' frustration in their talk of cases. Such talk does not translate in any direct way into practice. In order to gain access to the detailed personal information their work depends on, practitioners have to withhold judgement on the moral worth of their clients (Pithouse, 1987). To blame them directly is counterproductive, and women confronted in the heat of a worker's anxiety with no consideration for their own feelings rarely confided in social workers again. In practice the expectations social workers set for mothers depended more on the alternatives they had available for children than on any theoretical model of child sexual abuse (Hooper, 1990).

Mothers experienced the medical discourse in other ways than through their contact with agencies, however, through its influence on lay understandings of child sexual abuse, on which they also drew in order to make sense of their experience. Women who discover that their children have been sexually abused, especially by their own partner, face a situation of severe loss and confusion, in which many former assumptions about their worlds are overturned. In their search for meaning they are both vulnerable to and often resist available definitions of their roles.

Perhaps the most popular definition of mothers' roles in medical discourse is now the idea that there is a 'cycle of abuse' between mothers and daughters. The thesis of 'intergenerational transmission' is based on limited evidence but fits neatly within a family-systems perspective, legitimating professional intervention, and frequently making the abuser himself invisible. For mothers, 'cycle of abuse' theories have a subjective appeal in the 'why me? why her?' stage of coming to terms with loss, and one which carries strong risks, particularly where the guilt often felt in response to childhood sexual abuse is still unresolved. The following account illustrates this:

> I . . . thought to myself well maybe it was something that I did in my life, something bad, you know really bad that I'd done and she was being punished for it . . . all sorts of things went through my mind, I thought perhaps that it was because of when my father was abusing me, there were times when I actually enjoyed it.

While their own histories of abuse could cause extra distress, however, women also saw them positively as a resource, sometimes actively searching memory for experiences of their own that would help them understand those of their children.

Other components of the medical model also influenced women. The idea that abusers were 'sick' diminished their responsibility, since illness is generally regarded as outside the individual's control, and not deserving of blame (see Cornwell, 1984). It also implies the possibility of cure. To be an effective ally to a child requires attributing responsibility clearly to the offender, and those women who did so rejected such explanations, adopting an explicitly moral discourse involving conscious action ('He knew what he was doing') and personal responsibility ('old enough to know right from wrong'). Similarly, the idea that sexual problems in their own relationships might explain the abuser's actions both diminished his responsibility and could cause devastating guilt for mothers, unless it was accompanied by a clear sense of their own right to sexual autonomy.

Child-protection discourse

The medical discourse is not insignificant in its impact on either social workers or mothers. However, in their practice social work agencies draw more, I would argue, on a child-protection discourse which is preoccupied not with causality but with parental responsibility. A phrase reminiscent of the earliest and most misogynistic of advocates of family dysfunction, that mothers are crucial or central, recurs in child-protection discourse but for different reasons, that as primary carers, mothers are usually the key person in preventing further abuse and thus obviating the need to receive the child into care. The role and responsibility accorded mothers in this discourse raises more complex issues for feminists, at least if the need for some social control role on behalf of children is accepted (see Gordon, 1986).

There are two main problems with the way in which parental responsibility is commonly attributed to women. First, the problem is that women are commonly accorded *sole* responsibility for the welfare of children (not that they bear *any* responsibility), and further, that they lack the resources to exercise it effectively. Motherhood is thus characterised by 'powerless responsibility' (Rich, 1977). The implicitly gendered assumptions that underlie discussion of parental responsibilities are illustrated by the argument of Bentovim and colleagues that: 'a parent who knows that the other parent is in a state of depression, anger or frustration and leaves that parent to care for the child . . . indicates a failure in sharing responsibility' (Bentovim *et al.*, 1987: 29). This clearly means mothers leaving depressed fathers. If fathers who left depressed mothers to care for children were cause for state intervention, social services departments (SSDs) would be swamped.

Second, parents are commonly presented as an indivisible unit with identical interests, obscuring the conflicts between them. The Department of Health, for example, suggests that showing remorse and taking responsibility for abuse are positive indicators in the assessment of parents (DoH, 1988a). For a non-abusing mother in cases of child sexual abuse, the opposite is more likely to be the case. Despite evidence that the battering of women frequently precedes both physical and sexual child abuse (see Truesdell et al., 1986; Stark and Flitcraft, 1988; Hooper, 1990), this rarely merits a mention in the mainstream child-abuse literature or policy debate. While both women and children often seek help from agencies to control the more powerful members of the household, official discussion of the social control role of social work constructs it as one-way, between the state and the family as a unit, and in practice the burden commonly falls on women.

Consequently, women in my study who sought help when their children were sexually abused sometimes received little but surveillance of themselves in return. Where they had been victimised themselves, an approach to authority by social workers which failed to disaggregate parents was particularly counter-productive. Women used to resisting their partner's control and fighting to retain some of their own simply adopted similar strategies, focusing on 'beating the system', when another authority stepped in to set rules for them. Children, too, already used to seeing their mothers powerless, are likely to have this perception reinforced in witnessing such encounters with professionals, increasing their own insecurity. The control role was not always unwelcome to mothers, but they wanted it used to back up their own efforts rather than turned against them. Their criticisms were of the failure of social workers to exercise authority at the appropriate time and with the appropriate person, and the tendency to accord them greater powers than they had to control abusive men themselves.

Despite these common problems, the discourse of child protection could be used to empower women, since local authorities and social workers have considerable discretion to negotiate their policies and practices within the broad framework set out by central government. Both mothers' and social workers' accounts of the child protection register illustrated this. All local authorities are required to hold a register, listing children who are known to have been abused or are thought to be at risk of abuse. There has been much confusion about the exact purpose of registers, and decisions to place children's names on them are often inconsistent (Corby, 1987). It is generally assumed that they are stigmatising to parents, and suggestions have been made that they be scrapped. However, registration has variable meanings, both to social workers and mothers. Social workers did not perceive the decision simply as a bureaucratic one, but one made within the context of negotiating a complex set of relationships. Thus decisions were sometimes influenced by the message that registration might give to the mother (the possibility of either damaging an existing relationship of co-operation or of motivating an improved one), to the child (showing a complaint had been taken seriously), or to a new authority when a family was moving (attempting to ensure the allocation of a social worker). Some mothers certainly did experience registration as unjust, especially where the child had no further contact with the abuser, saying, for example, that it was like a criminal conviction against them. Others, however, did not, seeing it positively as giving either entitlement to priority help, or backing to exclude an abusive partner from the house.

Judicial discourse

Judicial discourse involves further constructions of women whose children are sexually abused, as sources of domestic stress (primarily through the breakdown of sexual relationships), the financial dependants of men and agents of informal control, which are crucial to approaches to offenders. The Parole Board for 1968 advocated a welfare approach to incest offenders on the assumption that inadequate sexual relationships with their wives were at root (Bailey and McCabe, 1979), implicitly endorsing men's right to sexual satisfaction within the family. Sentencing practice reinforces traditional family structures by its use both of sexual estrangement and a continuing marital relationship as mitigating factors. Thus, fathers are returned to the position of power in families which is at the root of incestuous abuse (Mitra, 1987). The case for non-custodial sentences with conditions of treatment is also based to a large extent on the effects of family breakup and the loss of a breadwinner on 'the family' (Glaser and Spencer, 1990).

In this debate women are presented as naturally, or at least happily, dependent and hence invariably resistant to the prosecution of their husbands. In my study, however, while fear of losing a breadwinner was an issue for some women, inhibiting reporting, for others fear that no effective legal action would be taken was the more important factor increasing their sense of isolation and powerlessness in the family. The possibility of prosecution had both negative and positive meanings, the most important of the latter being the clear message it gave about the individual responsibility of the abuser, and an opportunity to discover their own capacity for independence. In practice, the effectiveness of non-custodial alternatives for offenders rests on the informal controls operated by the family (i.e. women) as well as court orders on treatment and residence (Wolf *et al.*, 1988), although this role is often invisible in debates.

CONCLUDING REMARKS

I have aimed in this chapter to highlight some of the varying ways in which responsibilities have been attributed to women and girls in constructions of child sexual abuse, both at different periods of history and in competing discourses. Over the period considered, from the 1870s to the present, the greater recognition of children's needs alongside a recurring reluctance to consider collective or male responsibility for meeting them, has resulted in increased expectations of mothers. Women have gained rights as well as responsibilities over this period of course, to political citizenship, greater access to education and paid employment, divorce and a minimal level of welfare provision. While they are therefore somewhat less subject to the control of individual men in the household, their move into the public sphere has been accompanied by continued subordination within it (Walby, 1990). Women's disadvantage in the labour market and responsibility for child care (before and after divorce) mean divorce carries a high risk of poverty. Yet 'reasonable parental care', as expressed in the Children Act 1989, is defined according to expectations of 'the average or reasonable parent', abstracted from social context, who must, if unable to meet their child's needs themselves, seek help from others who can (DoH, 1989b). If women are to meet these expectations when a partner abuses their child, then the economic dependence which inhibits them both from stopping such abuse themselves and from seeking help must be addressed, and when they do seek help, services which meet their own needs and their children's must be available.

In conclusion, I want to comment briefly on the impact of feminist definitions of child sexual abuse on current policy. There are increasing attempts to sever family-systems thinking from its preoccupation with causality and its reactionary sexual politics, and to integrate it with feminist analyses (see e.g. Masson and O'Byrne, 1990). The DoH no longer attributes incestuous abuse to 'distorted family relationships' (DHSS, 1988) but cautiously accepts the need for further explanatory frameworks (DoH, 1989a). At the same time as the claims of family therapists are being modified, however, wider social anxieties about 'family breakdown' encourage resort to its practices. The danger is that the use of such practices will be driven more by the New Right's attempt to buttress the traditional family than any evidence of their effectiveness in preventing abuse, and attention diverted from alternative strategies to reduce the social and economic disadvantages that family breakdown brings for women and children.

The DoH has also adopted the concept of non-abusing parents (usually mothers), who 'may need help to adjust to the changes in their lives' (DoH, 1989a: 29), and the recommendation that abusing men should be excluded from the home in preference to removing children into care. Here, there is a danger that in the current political context, the changes for which feminists have campaigned may have perverse effects. Where SSDs are starved of resources and collective responsibility for child care is minimal, the designation of women as non-abusing parents may facilitate their definition simply as resources for their children rather than women with their own needs, and the exclusion of abusing men may increase women's responsibilities while depleting their resources. To turn such strategies to the empowerment of women and children demands their location within a broader programme of social change.

NOTES

1 The figures produced by the NSPCC, based on a sample of registers covering about 10% of the child population in England and Wales, show that the number of children on registers more than doubled from 1983 to 1987, and the proportion of these who had been sexually abused increased from 5% in 1983 to 28% in 1987 (S.J. Creighton and P. Noyes, *Child Abuse Trends in England and Wales 1983–1987*, London: NSPCC, 1989).

2 NSPCC *Annual Reports* 1893–94, 1906–07, 1907–08, 1908–09, 1910–11, 1912–13, 1913–14, 1914–15 and 1918–19.

3 The Home Office had issued a circular in 1926 backing some of the recommended changes in police and court practice, but allowing discretion for varying local circumstances.

4 See *Report of the Joint Committee on Sexual Offences*, December 1935; *Sexual Offences against Young Persons: Memorandum for Magistrates*, December 1935; *Memorandum on 'The Need for a Medical–Mental Examination of Persistent Sexual Offenders'* by Dr Gillespie, December, 1935. These, the minutes of the Joint Committee and correspondence concerning it, on which this chapter draws, are located in the NVA archives, Fawcett Library, London.

5 See *Report of the Royal Commission on the Care and Control of the Feeble-Minded*, vol. VIII, London: HMSO, 1908: pp. 120–1.

6 Miss E.H. Kelly, a member of the 1925 Committee and of the National Council of Women made this case. AMSH also claimed to have suggested it in 1918 (*The Shield*, Feb–Mar 1926).

7 *The Vote*, for example, carried a column entitled variously 'How Men Protect Women', 'How Some Men Protect Women', and 'The Protected Sex', which reported cases of violence against women and children and the paltry sentences which men commonly received for them.

8 Behlmer (1982) traces it back to 1816.

9 See Jeffreys (1982) for a review of these campaigns, and Bland (1983) for variations amongst Victorian feminists in attitudes to sex.

10 See discussion on 'The Problem of the Moral Pervert', reported in *Journal of the Institute of Hygiene*, April 1933: 236–8.

11 The Criminal Justice Act 1988 introduced an experimental scheme allowing children to give evidence in the Crown Court through a live, closed-circuit television link. Further changes have recently been proposed using video-recorded interviews, which would allow children to give evidence before the trial, thus avoiding the distress caused by long delays (Pigot Committee, *Report of the Advisory Group on Video Evidence*, London: Home Office, 1989). The Children Act 1989 also enabled civil proceedings relating to children to admit hearsay evidence and the unsworn evidence of a child.

12 See MacLeod (1982) for a review of these changes and their implications.

13 See London Borough of Brent, *A Child in Trust: Report of the panel of inquiry investigating the circumstances surrounding the death of Jasmine Beckford*, 1985; London Borough of Greenwich, *A Child in Mind: Protection of Children in a Responsible Society, The Report of the Comission of*

Inquiry into the circumstances surrounding the death of Kimberley Carlisle, 1987; and London Borough of Lambeth, *Whose Child? A Report of the Public Inquiry into the death of Tyra Henry*, 1987.

14 See Secretary of State for Social Services, *Report of the Inquiry into Child Abuse in Cleveland 1987*, London: HMSO, 1988.

Chapter 4

Women and late-nineteenth-century social work

Jane Lewis

The late-nineteenth century was marked by new efforts to regulate the behaviour of the urban working class by entering the homes of the people, with the result that working-class women were confronted with visitors of all kinds: school attendance officers, inspectors from the National Society for the Prevention of Cruelty to Children, parish visitors and, in the case of many of those applying for charitable relief, visitors from the Charity Organisation Society. Most of this activity was confined to the voluntary sector and was conducted by middle-class women, who dealt with working-class wives and mothers.

The nature of this form of personal social work has been the subject of considerable commentary and criticism by historians. First, there is the question of the motives of those undertaking it. Feminist historians have speculated on the self-interests of those involved. Anne Summers (1979) has suggested that the middle-class woman used social work as virtually the only available bridge to the public world of work and citizenship. The work was (usually) unpaid and represented an acceptable extension of women's domestic concerns. Thus, in Summers's analysis, these women left their own homes in order to inform working-class women of the merits of good housewifery and motherhood. There were certainly women who used philanthropic visiting of this kind as a stepping stone to other sorts of work. Perhaps most famous was Beatrice Webb, who began work outside the home as a social worker/rent collector, but who soon left the predominantly women's world of practical social work for the more male-dominated field of social investigation. Others went from philanthropic work into suffrage activities.[1] But many more remained committed to individual social work with the poor. They may well have welcomed the work as a satisfying and acceptable outlet for their energies; Martha Vicinus (1986) has argued convincingly that social work both offered a challenge and provided a sense of community, especially to the unmarried women undertaking it. But the work was often far from congenial. Beatrice Webb certainly detested the smells, the dirt and the brutality, and yet large numbers of women engaged in it for long periods of their adult lives. It seems that their commitment (at least in so far as can be determined from the work of the leading proponents of personal service) went rather deeper than self-interest.

A majority of historians have sought to locate women's early social work in the context of the growth of the state and the perceived shift from 'individualism' to 'collectivism'. Without closely investigating the ideas of the proponents of social work (who were predominantly women), the tendency has been to characterise their work as an exercise in regulating and disciplining the poor.[2] A few (mainly American) women historians, interested predominantly in the practice of voluntary work, both social and administrative, in institutions – in workhouses, schools and hospitals – have taken a rather different view. They have suggested that such women effectively improved the conditions of inmates and have characterised their work as 'domesticating politics'.[3] This may be a rather optimistic view in that both the motives and practice of those involved in this more broadly based social work varied considerably. But there is probably more justification for giving the work of women in social administration a better press in terms of its outcome, than individual social work. It is striking that in the early-twentieth century working-class women seem to have welcomed the opportunity to visit the new infant welfare centres, often called 'schools for mothers', where they could take advantage of the information offered about babies' health and ignore more prescriptive advice on household management, but to have shown less warmth towards the uninvited health visitor (see Mitchell, 1968; Lewis, 1980).

Nevertheless, the ideas and practice of early individual social work are more complicated than the simple idea of 'women controlling women' would suggest. The work was certainly grounded individualism and aimed to foster independence of both state and charitable relief by encouraging family members to fulfil their (gendered) obligations towards one another: men to take responsibility for breadwinning and women for the good management of the household. But 'individualism' represented a method of dealing with the problem of poverty as well as the goal of self-maintenance. Those women involved in the house-to-house visiting of the poor believed in treating the needs of individuals in a holistic fashion within the context of the family, as well as in getting the family to stand on its own feet.

This chapter provides an analysis of the ideas and work of two women who were perhaps the most influential proponents of individual social work during the second half of the nineteenth century, Octavia Hill and Helen Bosanquet.[4] Octavia Hill was a founder member of the Charity Organisation Society (COS), which was the most influential organisation promoting the ideas of 'scientific' charity,[5] and began her work of housing management in the mid-1860s, holding firmly to the importance of quiet, detailed, individual social work until her death in 1912. Helen Dendy was also a pillar of the COS and worked as one of its district secretaries in the early 1890s until her marriage to the Idealist philosopher, Bernard Bosanquet, in 1894. She was far more eager to theorise her work than Octavia Hill, who dismissed most efforts at analysis as so much 'windy talk', and she achieved considerable influence in the training of social workers, both through her editorship of the *Charity Organisation Review*, from 1909 to 1912, and her books on the lives of the poor and the problem of poverty.

These women were inspired to social action in different ways, Octavia Hill by a strong Christian impulse, and Helen Bosanquet more by the tenets of Idealist philosophy. But they both saw individual social work in the context of the family as the means to social progress. They emphasised the need to empathise with the poor, and to know and understand the fabric of their lives and hence their problems; they achieved a particularly sympathetic understanding of the position of working-class wives. The aim of the social worker was to work with the poor family and not to dictate to it. However, the aim was also in the final analysis to change the habits of family members, such that the family unit became self-maintaining. But the approach was, at least in theory, not so much disciplinary as designed to achieve a measure of empowerment. All this is to present late-nineteenth-century social work in a significantly different light from most historians.[6]

Nevertheless, there is little evidence as to how the idea of social work was carried out in practice and virtually nothing to tell us about what went on when the social worker met the client.

In practice the work may well have fallen considerably short of the ideal. Charity Organisation Society visitors were instructed to investigate the character of the applicant for relief and if he or she were deemed to be 'deserving' (a category relabelled 'helpable' during the 1890s), the visitor would undertake casework with the family. The aim was to enable the family to become self-sustaining: employment would be sought, patterns of thrift encouraged, the help of relatives enlisted. Only as a last resort would material relief be given. These ideas about the proper way in which to deal with the poor achieved widespread influence. They filtered into the work of parish visitors, too, who, even if they did not adhere strictly to COS principles, at least felt a twinge of guilt about the demoralising effects they might produce by giving out coal tickets or bread too freely. In the case of Octavia Hill's rent collectors, the principles were followed strictly and the collection of rent served as the occasion for personal social work. The collectors advised tenants who were experiencing financial problems as a result of unemployment or illness, or whose children's behaviour was giving rise to concern, thus helping to ensure that rent was paid regularly. But there is evidence of considerable tension in the work of both Hill and Bosanquet between the desire to 'know' and work with the poor on the one hand, and to change their ways on the other, and it is likely that the practice of their less-well-trained followers failed to live up to the theory on a number of counts.

However, the late-nineteenth-century female proponents of social work were by no means solely the reactionary handmaidens of classical political economy. Their holistic approach to the problems of poor families meant that they shared common ground with other female social investigators such as the Fabian Women's Group in terms of their qualitative analysis of the fabric of working-class women's lives, even though they differed radically in their opposition to state intervention. They opposed the idea that the study of poverty should become the study of aggregates (in the manner of Charles Booth and Benjamin Seebohm Rowntree's study of poverty in London and York, respectively), and they insisted on the voluntary nature of social work as a means of middle-class women fulfilling their obligations as citizens to serve others, thereby extending the possibility of an active citizenship to the poor, including working-class women. In the histories of social policy, which have tended to focus on the growth of the state, their contribution has been overlooked, as Prochaska (1988) has pointed out. More seriously still, their ideas were also lost within the bureaucracy of the welfare state, for while they came to occupy paid positions in social work, policy was made by a civil service that was almost entirely male in its upper echelons.

In the scramble to wash the charity and hence, it was believed, the stigma out of welfare provision, social work was divorced from social theory and ideas as to the importance of social participation were separated from the provision of an adequate standard of material wellbeing, which became the sole goal of the welfare state.

THE IDEA OF PERSONAL SOCIAL WORK

The mainspring of social action that Octavia Hill most freely acknowledged was that of duty, which was inspired above all by F.D. Maurice, the Christian Socialist. Maurice deplored the Utilitarian's pursuit of self-interest, stressing instead the importance of unselfish behaviour. The idea of the importance of self-giving as a manifestation of Christian obligation was central to many Victorian women social reformers. While it often involved a measure of self-sacrifice, it was not about self-denial, for only through giving to others would joy and happiness be achieved. To the end of the nineteenth century, duty would remain one of the chief organising principles behind the idea of women's mission to women, whether to poor mothers, or to prostitutes (Burdett Coutts, 1893).

Octavia Hill believed that all Christians were obliged to try to do the right thing. In 1873, she wrote to Henrietta Barnett, who had been one of her best rent collectors: 'I fight so desperately to be right, to see right, to do right'.[7] Above all, she believed that if everyone sincerely pursued 'right action', searching his or her conscience as to the path of duty, good would prevail. No one could be sure of doing right, nor could anyone impose an obligation on another person, the impetus for service and right action had to come from within each individual and be sincerely 'felt'.

The Christian duty to give of oneself was the same for men and women. However, tasks were clearly gendered. Frank Prochaska (1980) has observed the way in which men controlled finances and committees in the world of nineteenth-century charity, while women raised funds through bazaars and balls, and visited the poor. Similarly, Seth Koven (1987) has described how in the work of the London settlements, women tended to undertake personal visiting, became school board managers and ran schemes such as the Children's Country Holidays Fund, moving eventually into professional social work, while men concentrated more on lecturing, social investigation and local politics, often moving eventually into positions of power and influence as civil servants and politicians. F.D. Maurice (1893: 56) insisted that the roles of men and women in wider society should reflect the proper relationships between husbands and wives. Women's part was to cultivate 'the feelings which embrace and comprehend truth', while men cultivated 'the understandings which were destined to supply us with the outward and visible expression of it'. He invited middle-class women to consider how they might go to 'poor creatures as woman to woman' in order to minister to their 'diseased and anxious minds and to extend sympathy to calm their perturbed spirits' (Maurice, 1855: 55, 89–90). In Octavia Hill's view, women's duty lay in doing detailed, patient, gentle work in the homes of the poor, which had the benefit of coming closest to women's family duties in both its nature and scale.

Hill regarded individual work as the only lasting way of effecting social change: 'my only notion of reform is that of living side by side with people, till all that one believes becomes clear to them' (Maurice, 1928: 211). She profoundly distrusted systems and bureaucratic machinery and feared that working on a larger scale would mean working for a system: 'I would rather work in the unsought-after, out-of-sight places, side by side with my fellow workers, face to face with tenants than in the conspicuous forefront of any great movement'.[8]

The key to changing the behaviour of the poor lay in strengthening 'character', which was why such importance was attached to individual social work. As Stefan Collini (1985) has pointed out, the idea of character depended on a prior notion of duty and invocations of character 'in fact presupposed an agreed moral code'. Helen Bosanquet was just as preoccupied with the importance of weak character and bad habits as determinants of poverty. Indeed, both Octavia Hill and Helen Bosanquet have been accused of ignoring the structural causes of poverty and of adhering to the ideas of the classical economists, who believed that destitution was the result of individual moral failure. Historians have tended to perceive late-nineteenth-century individual social work as, at best, a futile and misguided attempt to solve the problem of poverty, which in fact demanded the kind of structural reform and state intervention that both Hill and Bosanquet abhorred.[9] At worst, the work has been judged as an effort to discipline the poor, leaving their real material needs for relief unmet. But this is to ignore the way in which its proponents conceived of the aims of individual social work.

Hill insisted that the aim was to do more than simply investigate as to whether an applicant for relief was of good character and therefore deserving of relief:

By knowledge of character more is meant than whether a man is a drunkard or a woman is dishonest, it means knowledge of the passions, hopes and history of people; where the temptation will touch them, what is the little scheme they have made of their lives, or would make, if they had encouragement, what training long past phases of their lives may have afforded; how to move, touch, teach them.

(Maurice, 1913: 258)

Hill insisted on the importance of knowing the whole person, claiming proudly and in terms that ran counter to the growing statistical movement, that 'my people are numbered, not merely counted, but known man, woman and child' (Hill, 1869: 224). The number of people she and her fellow workers could know was inevitably small, and anticipating criticism of the scale of her work, she demanded only whether the mass of people were not 'made up of many small knots'. All that was needed were armies of workers prepared to approach the poor in a new way. Hill's aim was to restore people to independence; to increase their self-respect and enable them to lead a 'better' life.

Helen Bosanquet, who did not share Hill's impatience with attempts to 'theorise' social work, elaborated these fundamental principles more fully. Her inspiration to social action came from political theory and Idealism rather than Christianity, but she shared Octavia Hill's conviction that the middle-class person desiring to do something about the condition of the poor must think through his or her actions from beginning to end and be prepared to take responsibility for exerting influence over the life of another. She also shared Octavia Hill's aim to do detailed long-term work with a family until its independence of outside material relief was assured and it was placed in a position where its members might become 'active citizens'. In Bosanquet's analysis, empowering the poor such that they were enabled actively to participate in society was the first priority, and material relief the second.

Bosanquet also stressed the importance of 'developing character', but this meant considerably more than an injunction to self-help. 'Ethical', as opposed to 'atomic', individualism involved the development of a more complete human nature, part of which required (in the same manner as Christian duty) the individual to fulfil his obligations to his fellow men. The poor should not be told to pull themselves up by their boot straps and be left to their own fate, but rather helped and restored to full citizenship. Helen Bosanquet pointed out that the lives of the rich as much as those of the poor could be 'one incoherent jumble from beginning to end', exhibiting 'the same self-indulgence, the same eager devotion to trifles and absorption in the interests of the moment' (Bosanquet, 1903: 51; Dendy, 1895a). To the extent that she insisted that all people were equally capable of developing or failing to develop character, her formulation was essentially democratic.

The task of the social worker was to repair the client's will and to build character. The first step to creating a purposeful and active citizen was to understand the client's perceptions of his or her condition: to work out why the client saw things in the way that he/she did, to appreciate his/her values and then to work to change bad habits. In elaborating this approach, Bosanquet turned not to the 'dismal science' of nineteenth-century classical economics, but rather to the fledgling discipline of psychology, from which she took the idea that human beings could be distinguished from the lower animals by their progressive wants. Bad habits would impede the progressive search for 'a higher standard' of life, which manifested itself, for example, in the desire for more living space and a more respectable neighbourhood (Bosanquet 1898a; 1903).

Both Hill and Bosanquet believed that the efforts of social workers should be concentrated on the family, which had greatest influence in the formation of good or bad habits. In particular, the family occupied a special place in Bosanquet's arguments regarding human motivation and behaviour. It was above all the primary institution in which character was developed and in which co-operative individuals and rational citizens were produced. In Bosanquet's last major book, *The Family* (1906), which in many ways represented the culmination of her thinking, she argued that the Family (always capitalised) was the fundamental social unit. Conceptualising it as a biological unit, Bosanquet portrayed the family as a natural building block in the enlargement of the individual's self-awareness. 'Natural' affection between husband and wife and between parent and child ensured that homes became nurseries of citizenship. The family was thus seen as the ethical root of a higher ethical state, mediating between the individual and the community. Bosanquet drew heavily on the work of the French sociologist, Frederick Le Play, who argued that 'good' family organisation was an essential factor contributing to the prosperity and contentment of a people. Where family members developed their sense of responsibility one to the other, Bosanquet argued, 'the Family presented itself as the medium by which the public interest is combined with private welfare'. In this analysis, social problems disappeared when the family was strong and effective; for example, old age pensions were unnecessary 'where the stable Family combines young and old in one strong bond of mutual helpfulness' (Bosanquet, 1906: 95, 99). Social workers would work with families in which interest in the welfare of each other was but poorly developed. By undertaking the work on the voluntary basis, the social worker would also strengthen her own character, thus deepening the ties of obligation within the community. As for the poor, Bosanquet believed as A.W. Vincent (1984) has pointed out, that 'charity' was not a gift but a right, although she also believed that the poor had the responsibility of submitting to social scientific casework investigation.

Bosanquet believed that personal social work would increase the common good through mutual service based on reason and love. The idea of charity as love was of course the essentially Christian ideal that inspired Hill. But Idealism pushed these ideas a stage further and characterised social work as combining faith in the world of facts with passion and wisdom. Social work practice combined careful investigation with love and the social worker strove for this through the 'completeness of casework'. The key was to seek an understanding of the individual in relation to his/her environment and then to work at the best method of promoting self-maintenance (Bosanquet, 1900).

IDEAL SOCIAL WORK PRACTICE: KNOWING, LOVING AND BEFRIENDING

Both Hill and Bosanquet stressed that the social worker should not merely dictate. Rather, she should know, love and befriend. Hill insisted that 'you cannot learn how to help a man, nor even get him to tell you what ails him, until you care for him'.[10] She urged all social workers to think of the poor as their husbands, sons and daughters, and to treat them accordingly. By making the effort to sympathise and to 'feel' with them, by entering thoroughly into their lives, the visitor would be able to befriend the visited, a necessary preliminary to effective individual work. With friendship came trust, the 'most beautiful trait' in the character of the poor, and then the visitor could be sure that the people were ready to listen; 'unpalatable truths' could only be conveyed from one friend to another. Henrietta Barnett (1881) referred to friendship as 'our weapon', and as Anthony Wohl (1971) has observed, it was perhaps easier to gain entry to a working-class home as a 'friendly visitor' than as a paid official. Certainly the women's sanitary association thought so and eagerly promoted the woman visitor as the 'mother's friend' (Davies, 1988). However, Hill deplored any idea of 'friendly inspection' as something bound to subvert natural friendship and trust. In her evidence to the 1885 Royal Commission on Housing, she rejected the idea of inspection, strongly favoured by some other witnesses, because in her experience the poor dreaded it (C. 4402; Q. 8901–5). Certainly, popular dislike of the 'kid-catcher' (school attendance officer) and the 'cruelty man' (the National Society for the Prevention of Cruelty to Children's inspector) was strong, and there is clear evidence of a more general working-class dislike of inquisitorial and stigmatising welfare in the late-nineteenth and early-twentieth centuries (Thane, 1984).

It is easy to criticise Hill's notion of building friendship and trust as naïve. But she would have insisted that her particular mix of business philanthropy protected her rent collectors from just this sort of criticism. They visited for a purpose and trust grew not just out of friendship but out of the fulfilment of the mutual obligations of landlord and tenant, that is, out of the business relationship. In her evidence to the 1885 Royal Commission on Housing, she referred to the way in which her philanthropy, unlike the paternalism of the old Lady Bountiful, was geared to achieving the fulfilment of obligations on the part of rich and poor in crowded urban slums (C. 4402; Q. 8986). The vehicle for the expression of these obligations was the right use of money. In her work of housing management, the lady managers (on behalf of a landlord) kept accurate rent books and accounts, carried out repairs and made sure that the property paid its way, while tenants were obliged first and foremost to pay their rent. Individual work with the poor took place on the occasion of paying rent. Ellen Chase (1929), an American who worked with Hill for many years in Deptford, the area in which Hill experienced the most difficulty in her work, wrote simply and without comment of friendship growing out of the business relationship.

Hill was convinced that the regular visits of rent collectors would eventually result in better habits among tenants. Land-ladies, she felt, were a more influential force than teachers in the lives of the poor (Hill, 1875). She encouraged her rent-collector social workers to take an interest in every detail of the tenants' lives; everything was a part of life and therefore mattered and people could only be understood as wholes. The main work of the rent collector was to bring order and cleanliness and quiet out of chaos and dirt and to raise the 'standard' of the tenants. Collecting worked on two fronts, to encourage both changes in personal habits and a corporate sense of belonging in the dwellings. Hill's best reward was when her mother reported to her that a tenant was grateful that her court had become 'so quiet and respectable' (Maurice, 1913: 387). Rent collectors got to know their families. They made careful investigations, just as did Charity Organisation Society visitors, of employers, kin and previous landladies before taking on a new tenant, and they attended to repairs, undertaking 'indestructible repairs on the drains first' (Hill, 1875: 84). The difficulties of financing and carrying out repairs in what were very run-down buildings were enormous, but after some initial hiccoughs, it would seem that Hill maintained a better standard of basic repairs than have many local authorities in the post-war period. Rent collectors also judiciously gave out scrubbing work in the buildings to a deserving widow or to a girl too young for domestic service; arranged a country holiday for a child, a sewing class or a party or excursion for a group of tenants. When the most respectable member of a court died, Hill wrote of the importance of leaving his friends to help his widow, but of then stepping in 'with strong quiet lasting aid and help to earn or something of that kind'.[11] Collectors also made sure that respectable working people did not have to suffer drunken neighbours and they endeavoured to resolve long-standing quarrels, for example, between women over the use of a wash tub. Hill was fond of describing the work as quiet, detailed and continuous:

> for the work is one of detail . . . day after day the work is one of such small things, that if one did not look beyond and through them they would be trying – locks to be mended, notices to be served, the missing shilling of the week's rent to be called for three or four times, petty quarrels to be settled, small rebukes to be spoken, the same remonstrances to be made again and again.
>
> (Hill, 1875: 105)

At an appropriate moment, the social worker would be able to suggest to the tenant that another room be taken, thus encouraging tenants always to aspire to the 'next standard'. Because she believed that tenants would raise their standards but slowly, Hill opposed the new, model dwellings with their self-contained flats which did not afford the possibility of tenants renting another room. Similarly, she believed that amenities had to be kept basic. Appliances and facilities could only be improved gradually. Beatrice Webb passionately denounced Hill's ideas as to what standard of amenity was appropriate for poor tenants. On the other hand, Hill's repeated reference to her class of tenants as 'destructive' was not without foundation; vandalism was a major problem. She did not deny the importance of gradually improving amenities and was a lifelong campaigner for introducing as much natural beauty, light and aim into the slums as possible. She wrote passionately in her turn about watching the air disappear from London courts with the continual advance of speculative builders: 'This is different from reason and science: this is life, this is pain' (Hill, 1888: 181). She supported the efforts to decorate public buildings, and she spent a large amount of time soliciting voluntary subscriptions to collectively purchase anything from open spaces the size of Parliament Hill Fields to brightly coloured tiles for the outside wall of one of her properties, which spelled a suitably uplifting message: 'Every house is builded by some man but he that built all things is God'. She made several attempts to fence the garden of her first set of properties and then to plant it, describing her struggle in terms of a battle for order:

> You know something of how hard I worked for it [her first row of London houses] long ago; my difficulties in building the wall, and in contending with the dirt of the people, how gradually we reduced it to comparative order, have paved it, lighted it, supplied water cisterns, raised the height of the rooms, built a staircase, balcony and additional storey, how Mr. Ruskin had live trees planted for us and creepers, and by his beautiful presents of flowers helped to teach our people to love flowers. You know or can imagine, how dear the place is to me.
>
> (Maurice, 1913: 293)

The imposition of order was thus not entirely a matter of disciplining tenants. Hill's own efforts were substantial.

Both Hill and Bosanquet focused on the female members of the family as a focus for social work and both were sympathetic to the position of the working-class wife. Hill wrote to her cousin, Mary Harris, that she deplored the way in which haggard, careworn women tenants came 'cringing down' to her. She felt that she wanted to say: 'Don't treat me with such respect. In spirit I bow down to you, feeling that you deserve reverence, in that you have preserved any atom of God's image of you degraded and battered as you are by the world's pressure' (Maurice, 1928: 190). In common with many late-nineteenth-century social investigators and commentators, Bosanquet observed the importance of the working-class wife in securing the welfare of the family. Her skill as a household manager would determine the level of comfort achieved by families with a similar income and at a similar stage of family building. She believed the majority took their responsibilities for their children seriously. Only a minority could be considered wilfully neglectful through drink or gossip. In her first book she spoke of their 'patient endurance, unceasing sacrifice and terrible devotion' (Bosanquet, 1896: 102, 107). Their role was crucial in that they were the most strategic figures in the process of developing character in the next generation: 'If the husband is the heart of the Family, the wife is the centre' (Bosanquet, 1906: 279). Bosanquet's sympathy for the working woman's efforts to do well by her children sprung both from the belief that they were well intentioned but ignorant, and from a latent feminist understanding that they were by no means the arbiters of their own fate.

She recognised the difficulty of budgeting on an irregular income and of avoiding the temptation of credit. She demonstrated a thorough knowledge of the options of borrowing, pawning and delaying payment, and her estimate of the rates of interest involved – 24 per cent for pawnbrokers and up to 400 per cent for private money lenders – have been confirmed by a recent historical study (Bosanquet, 1898a; Tebbut, 1983). She knew how it was that a costermonger's business practices forced him to use credit, and how a housewife might use the pawnbroker as a way of 'equalising income'. She also appreciated the problems of cooking on an open fire and condemned the typical ignorance of the well-meaning philanthropist of the limitations on the choice of menus. And she realised how early marriage and frequent pregnancy could erode rather than develop maternal instinct. Watching a working-class wedding, she reflected on

> the light hearted way in which they take this step. For the girls especially it means burdens which seem almost too heavy to be born – of care and sickness and poverty, of hopeless squalor and unceasing toil, leading to premature old age or death. By the time they are 25 all the elasticity and vigour of youth are crushed out of them and those who maintain their self respect have nothing to look forward to but drudgery.
>
> (Dendy, 1895b: 76)

In writing of the working-class wife, Bosanquet was often uncharacteristically bleak. But her admiration for the heroic struggle mounted by so many working-class women caused her to believe that wives could nevertheless be educated to aim at a higher 'standard' for themselves and their families. 'Patient endurance' was also, she felt, accompanied all too often by 'patient unintelligence'. Where children were badly behaved, for example, she advised the social worker that 'the hard working mother of a large family is apt to lose sight of the fact that troublesomeness in children is often due to ill health which a wise and sympathetic visitor may be able to detect and check' (Bosanquet, 1898b: 15).

Significantly, she felt that of all women it was the working-class wife and mother who needed the vote, it would bring her to take more interest in the world around her and would give her more leverage in her profoundly unequal relationship with her husband. Bosanquet had no difficulty in accommodating the idea that women as rational creatures should seize every opportunity to widen their horizons, including the political; 'we all of us tread our daily round the better when there is at least one window through which we can look away to the hills'.[12]

Hill and Bosanquet were aware that social workers would experience difficulty in integrating the understanding they managed to achieve of the client's world and perceptions with work to change habits and cultivate higher aspirations. Hill was anxious to stress the importance of courtesy and respect in the dealings between her fellow workers and poor women. Maurice had also given considerable attention to the issue of communication between rich and poor, urging visitors to do as they would be done by and not to reprove or find fault, as well as being aware that the barriers to social intercourse might be different among working people. He warned that the destitute had for 'so long been used as anvils for other people to hammer out their own goodness on', that it would take time to put relations with the poor on a normal footing (Maurice, 1855: 279). Hill told her fellow workers that they must 'show the same respect for the privacy and independence (of the poor) and should treat them with the same courtesy that I should show towards other personal friends' (Hill, 1875: 77). How far this was followed, even to the extent of knocking on a door before entering is not clear, for the advice was repeated at frequent intervals by women social workers throughout the late-nineteenth and early-twentieth centuries, and still found a place in Emelia Kanthack's advice to health visitors, published in 1907.

In her turn, Bosanquet stressed that minds had to be prepared for new ideas and that what minds saw depended in some measure on what they already were. This, as she observed, was what made 'intercourse between people of different "upbringings" so difficult', and she warned that this 'should make us especially careful in placing our ideas before minds less developed (or differently developed) than our own, without making sure how they are interpreted' (Bosanquet, 1897: 273–4). One of the most important concerns of the late-Victorian middle class was the lack of communication between rich and poor, and both the Charity Organisation Society in its individual casework and the settlement movement aimed to bring the social classes back into contact. However, the task was found to be extraordinarily difficult. One of the chief refrains running through the works of early-twentieth-century social investigation, including that of Bosanquet, was the lack of understanding between classes (McKibbin, 1978). Inevitably, social workers identified the perceptions of the poor in relation to their own understanding of what was conducive to good character, and to this extent work with the poor slipped away from the idea of empowerment and towards social control.

THE REALITY OF SOCIAL WORK PRACTICE

Hill and Bosanquet's insistence on the importance of social workers reaching an understanding and appreciation of the values and ways of living of the poor was genuine. But there was, nevertheless, a clear set of beliefs and behaviours according to which the poor family would be judged. While some practices alien to the middle class, such as the willingness of working-class fathers to play with small children, were lauded, others were condemned as constituting bad habits. The proper fulfilment of the duties of husbands and wives was held to be particularly important. Women were obliged to be good household managers, because, as Bosanquet observed, the welfare of the family rested on them. Thus, while Bosanquet showed a sensitive understanding of the crucial role that pawnbroking played in balancing the working-class wife's housekeeping budget, she nevertheless felt obliged to condemn the practice and to urge the social worker to encourage the practice of thrift. Similarly, notwithstanding her concern to draw attention to the good qualities of the working-class husband and father, her primary concern centred on his willingness to provide. 'Natural' regard for his family's welfare was the primary impetus to the development of the adult male and his becoming a co-operative member of society:

Nothing but the considered rights and responsibilities of family life will ever rouse the working man to his full degree of efficiency, and induce him to continue working after he has earned sufficient to meet his own personal needs. The Family in short, is from this point of view, the only known way of ensuring, with any approach to success, that one generation will exert itself in the interests and for the sake of another, and its effect upon the economic efficiency of both generations is in this respect alone of paramount importance.

(Bosanquet, 1906: 222)

A number of tensions arose between the theory of social work practice and its reality. Both Helen Bosanquet and Octavia Hill insisted that individual casework represented an opportunity to develop relations between rich and poor based on love and sympathy. But the desire to promote interaction between rich and poor as freely associating individuals with the aim of raising the standards and level of happiness of the poor was hard to achieve in practice and Bosanquet's writing on social work methods often revealed contradictions in her thinking about the way in which the rich were to approach and 'treat' the poor. 'Thorough charity' demanded scientific investigation of circumstances and character and inevitably represented a substantial intrusion into the privacy of the family, which Bosanquet also insisted was crucial to the development of true family feeling. She urged social workers to think carefully before assuming the 'heavy responsibility' of intervening in the lives of others, but nevertheless assumed that respectable people would not mind inquiries being made of friends, neighbours and employers about their circumstances and character (Dendy, 1893).

Setting questions for discussion by trainee social workers in 1912, Bosanquet posed two issues which remain relevant today:

1. What circumstances or conditions justify intervention in the private life of a family which has not offended against the law?
2. How far are we in danger of mistaking a mode of life which we should not take ourselves for one which must necessarily be put a stop to?[13]

With regard to the first issue Bosanquet advised social workers to 'see the head of the family before giving assistance (for instance in respect of a truant child) . . . he has the right to be consulted before we interfere with his duty of providing for his family. Often he will be found very much adverse to charity' (Bosanquet, 1898b: 21). In fact, the evidence suggests that working-class men and women were anxious to receive non-stigmatising, non-intrusive welfare.

Working women welcomed the advice offered by infant welfare clinics while continuing to be suspicious of the routine and uninvited visits by health visitors (Lewis, 1980). They were unlikely to have felt better disposed towards a voluntary worker whose job included 'scientific assessment', and who in all likelihood found Bosanquet's second question either extremely difficult to answer, or, worse, unworthy of serious attention.

Knowing and befriending the poor was difficult. Ideal social work practice required the social worker to work with the client until the latter found the strength to 'raise their standards' and meet their own needs. Such a method relied first, on the capacity to recognise sources of strength that might not be immediately apparent to the middle-class observer, and second, on a willingness to work with the poor rather than dictate to them. Both Bosanquet and Hill recognised these points, but were inclined to assert their authority when they considered it necessary. At the end of the day the extraordinary authority that many middle-class, female, volunteer social workers achieved derived in large measure from their social class. In a piece originally published in 1871, Hill (1875: 82) told the story of a woman tenant who locked her door and shouted loudly that she would not pay rent until something was done about her rooms. Hill reported that only 'perfect silence would make her voice drop lower'. In their dealing with the poor, middle-class women counted in large part on a measure of deferential behaviour towards well-spoken ladies. But in many cases, Hill's included, authority gained an additional edge because of the belief that it was literally God-given. In 1869 Hill described the 'awed sense of joy' she felt in taking over her first court and having 'the moral power to say, by deeds that speak louder than words, "where God gives me authority, this, which you in your own hearts know to be wrong shall not go on" ' (Hill, 1869: 220). Geoffrey Best's (1964: 480) judgement of the work of rent collection, reached some 25 years ago, seems most accurate in terms of its assessment of the outcome, if not the intention of the work: the poor would be helped if they would submit.

Hill, for example, found herself unable to allow the members of the Boys' Club that she ran in connection with one of her housing projects to open the club on Sundays. While she maintained that the club members were 'the best judges of their own affairs', and that she did not want to 'tyrannise', when push came to shove, respect for the members' autonomy was subordinated to her own sense of what was fit, and working with these tenants in a spirit of friendship gave way to the exercise of firm control.[14] Similarly, while Bosanquet urged social workers to appreciate that legitimate sources of happiness existed among working people that were alien to the middle-class experience, there were many occasions on which she showed a propensity to ignore her own teaching that all social classes and all individuals had a standard which must be slowly and painfully improved, preferring to impose standards of behaviour of her own. Thus meeting indoors was to be preferred to the tendency of working people to congregate on the street, and the female factory worker was to be 'taught' to buy warm underclothing rather than 'feathers and finery' (Dendy, 1895c: 42). Because higher standards were inevitably associated with those of the middle class, the tendency was to teach social workers that the poor looked at things differently; that they should look for the 'sunnier side' of the poor's behaviour; but should then set about teaching more acceptable practices. Thus the idea of working with the poor translated itself in practice into something rather more didactic. Despite deploring the way in which philanthropic ladies tended to treat the poor as dependent children, believing that this merely encouraged them to behave as such, Bosanquet nevertheless described the state of mind of poor and uneducated wives as being akin to that of an untrained child and advised social workers that they should be prepared to develop the 'qualities of capacity and foresight for lack of which, more than for lack of money, so many make failures of their lives' (Bosanquet, 1896: 140). In other words, the social worker must be prepared to think for the poor on the assumption that the world view of the social worker would make inherently better sense than that of the poor.

The major criticism levied at late-nineteenth-century social work has been that it failed to provide a solution to the problem of poverty. The social surveys of Charles Booth and Benjamin Seebohm Rowntree showed the dimensions of the problem to be vast; one-third of the population of both London and York were 'in poverty'. Even though Hill and Bosanquet recognised the need for 'armies of social workers', an individual solution to the problem of poverty was not possible and the Liberal Government of 1906–1914 used the government machinery so deplored by both Hill and Bosanquet to deal with the problems of particular groups, albeit only those considered more deserving. Thus children, the elderly and the regularly employed male worker were taken outside the poor law and offered school meals, pensions and national unemployment and health insurance respectively. There is little doubt but that social work could not serve to provide a vehicle for achieving social change as its proponents wished. This was recognised by early-twentieth-century social workers, who held to the ideal of voluntary personal service, while also demonstrating a willingness to co-operate with the state.

It is more difficult to arrive at a verdict on the nature of the social work that was advocated and practised in the late-nineteenth century. While the motives had as much to do with empowering the poor as active citizens as with imbuing them with middle-class values, which was to be achieved by knowing and befriending the poor rather than dictating to them, in practice most social workers probably found it hard either to appreciate the world view of the poor, or to love and befriend people whose lives appeared disordered and often brutal. Certainly, Beatrice Webb quickly gave up collecting rents in the mid-1880s and did not hide her revulsion from the dirt and decay in the tenements.[15] Yet it is likely that the kind of social work advocated by Hill and Bosanquet worked better in connection with rent collection than it did for the visitors who worked for the Charity Organisation Society among those declaring themselves destitute. The rent collector had more scope for 'preventive' work among people who had usually been chosen as tenants for their reliability. Rent collectors could help families to weather periods of misfortune and also offer a reasonable standard of repairs and maintenance services in return. It appears that tenancies in Hill's blocks were sought after and her housing-management failures were few. Beatrice Webb's vivid descriptions of the bleak conditions in the buildings she worked in may have had more to do with her middle-class sensibilities than with the standards of cleanliness and propriety *per se*, although it was all too easy for Hill's prescriptions as to the provision of only basic levels of amenities in the first instance to be interpreted meanly, just as it was for Bosanquet's ideas to be interpreted more in terms of the negative refusal of relief than of the positive long-term need for social work support.

Indeed, it is far from clear that the proponents of late-nineteenth-century social work were successful in their aim of empowering the poor. At best, the poorly trained, well-meaning, middle-class, female social workers may have ended up taking the more traditional Lady Bountiful approach'and giving or lending money, which gave the satisfaction of inducing gratefulness in the recipient. At worst, they may have denied material help while simultaneously failing to provide any other assistance. But from their close observation and sympathetic understanding of the poor, Hill and Bosanquet well understood that poverty was a more complicated issue than material deprivation alone. Those who, like Beatrice Webb, rejected the female world of social work and an individual approach to the problem of poverty became in turn committed to the imposition of an administrative solution from above and also failed to recognise the truth of Bosanquet's argument that cash benefits alone would not bring full citizenship.

Many historians have been ready to label late-nineteenth-century women's social work as an exercise in social control, and the debate about social work practice, a large part of which continues to be a matter of women dealing with women, still tends to be argued around the issue of 'women controlling women'. However the nineteenth-century reality was certainly more complicated than this, and while the methods of the early social workers may well have proved an inadequate vehicle for their ideas, those ideas nevertheless constituted an important approach to the treatment of poverty.

NOTES

1 For example, see the autobiography of Margaret Wynne Nevinson (1926).
2 The most powerful critique of the COS is that of Gareth Stedman Jones (1976). A much less subtle treatment is offered by Fido (1977). Stedman Jones (1977) also criticised casual use of the term 'social control'. In addition, F.M.L. Thompson (1981) condemned the way in which the concept allows little room for the possibility that working people themselves generated their own values and behaviours.
3 On Britain, see Hollis (1987). On the USA, see Baker (1984) and Scott (1984).
4 The material for the chapter comes from a larger piece of research on feminism and social problems in the lives of late-nineteenth and early-twentieth-century female social activists (Lewis, 1991).
5 The standard account of the work of the COS is that of Mowat (1961).
6 The major exception is the work of Vincent and Plant (1984), who have offered an important revisionary interpretation of the COS.

7 Octavia Hill to Henrietta Barnett, 26 December 1873, Coll. misc. 512, BLPES, LSE.
8 Octavia Hill, Letter to My Fellow Workers, 1882: p. 4, Hill Papers, Marylebone Public Library.
9 Many of the standard histories of the welfare state tend to this view, e.g. Fraser (1973).
10 Octavia Hill, Letter to My Fellow Workers, 1875: p. 7, Hill Papers.
11 Octavia Hill to Sidney Cockerell Sr, 6 May 1875, item 18, D. Misc. 84/3, Hill Papers.
12 Helen Bosanquet, 'A Reply to Mrs Humphry Ward', letter to *The Times*, 21 December 1911, Bosanquet Papers, Trunk 2, Pkt. K(6), Newcastle University Library.
13 Helen Bosanquet, 'Some Problems of Social Relief: How to Help Cases of Distress' (1912), np. Bosanquet Papers, Trunk 3.
14 Octavia Hill to Sidney Cockerell Sr, 13 April 1877, item 43, D. Misc. 84/3, Hill Papers.
15 Beatrice Webb, Diary TS, 7 November 1886, f. 745, BLPES, LSE.

Chapter 5

Producers of legitimacy
Homes for unmarried mothers in the 1950s

Martine Spensky

The numbers of women who came into the orbit of the Homes for
Unmarried Mothers in Britain in the 1950s might have been small
(only 20 per cent of all mothers in 1953) but studying them provides
information on complex social relations which coexisted and
interacted at that moment in history. This enquiry informs us
about the normative expectations placed on women in general,
since unmarried mothers are simply those who have deviated from
the dominant norm of reproductive behaviour assigned by gender
relations. It also throws light on other social relations, for example,
those of class and 'race'. Indeed, for the purposes of this paper it is
important that the concept 'illegitimacy' is not understood or read
only in its narrow legal sense. Rather, it should also be understood
as a social practice which is constructed as deviant by society at a
given period. In this instance the practice to which I refer is sexual
relations between people of different (i.e. inappropriate) social
classes or groups, one being treated as inferior to the other.

In order to analyse the function of these homes for unmarried
mothers it is useful, first, to analyse what unmarried motherhood
meant when compared to married motherhood. We will then
progress to see how it was dealt with in the main policy documents
which decided the fate of unmarried mothers for more than a
century, namely the New Poor Law legislation and the Beveridge
Report, which embodied all post-war welfare laws. Only then will
it be possible to ask the question whether the homes acted as a
social provision in favour of women, as a regulator of their
sexuality, or both.

UNMARRIED MOTHERS AS THE 'DELINQUENTS' OF GENDER RELATIONS AND OF THE SEXUAL DIVISION OF LABOUR

Until very recently, unmarried mothers were treated as the delinquents of gender relations. In a patriarchal society where power is in the hands of the fathers, a society where blood ties and property are privileged, it is important that fathers be sure of their paternity before they pass their names and property on to their sons. Their daughters are given to other families in order to produce sons. Until the end of the seventeenth century and even later, the father was thought to be the only biological producer of the child, while the mother was only considered to be a nurturing receptacle (Knibiehler and Fouquet, 1983). The possible introduction of a stranger into the well-to-do family was considered to be a felony to which the wife was the accomplice. Before women were able to control their reproduction – and even later, to a certain extent – gender relations were articulated around the control of women's bodies in order to ensure male reproduction. Women had to remain virgins till their wedding night, after which it was their marital duty to allow their husbands – and no one else – to have sex with them whenever they wished. Marriage gave women the status of respectability and some limited – but real – legal protection as dependants. The second best for women with regard to respectability was not to marry but to stay at home with their parents and look after them in their old age. They were supposed to remain virgins all their lives. Women's bodies were not their own. Men owned them on a private basis to ensure the continuation of their lineage through marriage, and collectively through the organisation of prostitution which provided them with non-procreative pleasure. The women who did not fall into the category of wives (private women) necessarily fell into the category of prostitutes (public women) who were not supposed to procreate.

The sexual division of labour reinforced the private/public dichotomy. In traditional society where a home-based economy was the norm, the sexual division of labour was not as clear cut as it became later, since all the people living under the same roof produced under the supervision of the head of the family. Women carried out the tasks linked to reproduction in addition to their productive work but the two spheres were not completely separate. With the advent of the wage system, the two spheres drifted apart, at least as far as representations and culture were concerned. In this system, reproduction and production were assigned different locations. Work was defined as paid work and work with no pay was considered non-work. Men were meant to work in production. They depended on their wages. Women were meant to deal only with reproduction. They depended on the wage of the man they lived with, whether they themselves were in paid employment or not. Women's low wages enforced their dependence on men. Therefore, the ideal family, in ideological terms, was – and still is – composed of a heterosexual couple, preferably married, raising children (Abbot and Wallace, 1989). The father is the head of the family. He gives his name to his wife and children and has access to the resources which he distributes according to his good will (and his abilities), sometimes very grudgingly (Pahl, 1980). A complex pattern of traditions and morality ensures the continuous control of women's sexuality, reinforced by the sexual division of labour which maintains their relationship of dependency.

This organisation of gender relations put the unmarried mother in a very awkward position. She had not kept her body intact until wedlock, she was not in a private and legitimate relationship and was consequently suspected of being a public woman: a prostitute. She availed herself of a body that did not belong to her, which was tantamount to stealing (Rowbotham, 1973). She started a female lineage which was obviously illegitimate since only male lineages can be legitimate. The law called her child 'filius nullius' (nobody's child) as late as 1968 (Teichman, 1982).

It was also referred to as *unwanted* as if all legitimate children had been wanted. Society certainly did not want illegitimate children. The unmarried mother's material life was – is – difficult as she depended on no man for her survival and had to be content with her wage, a woman's wage at that, which was not meant to keep a family. Since she was in the labour market full time, she was considered a 'bad mother' because English culture, which is the cradle of child psychology and psychoanalysis, has constructed motherhood as a full-time occupation. A good mother is supposed to devote herself entirely to her child. This was even more the case in the 1950s (Wilson, 1980).

I am very conscious of having painted an ahistorical picture of the construction of unmarried motherhood in relation to that of married motherhood. The situation of unmarried mothers has fluctuated, has altered, but all its elements remain just below the surface and become more or less conspicuous according to historical period and social class. It is obvious that the poor, who did not have any property, were more tolerant of unmarried mothers even if they were not as indifferent as has sometimes been claimed. Illegitimacy did not give a bad name to the family nor threaten property rights, which usually go together. However, the upkeep of a fatherless child, especially when the mother was young, fell to the maternal grandparents, putting the latter in a very difficult economic situation. The mother was often kept at home and the child was considered to be an additional financial burden. When the family could not afford it, she was thrown out of the house, more for economic than moral reasons. The middle-class unmarried mother was more harshly punished and was almost systematically thrown out, at least as long as she had not dumped the child somewhere and could not come back without anyone knowing about it. Middle-class parents watched over their daughters' sexuality, hoping other parents would do the same so that they could pass their name and property to their legitimate and biological grandchildren. Their sons were encouraged to play around with lower-class girls, considered to be bolder, while awaiting for the 'intact' bride of his own class who would beget legitimate children. The illegitimate children he might have visited upon the lower-class girl were not considered his by his family.

The Old Poor Laws gave the unmarried mother the right to name the father of her child who was compelled to give her an allowance. Bourgeois men were not as ready to recognise their illegitimate offsprings as the nobility had been in the old Feudal society (Teichman, 1982). In the preparatory debates of the Bastardy Clauses of the New Poor Law, the Commissioners voiced their fear of seeing lower-class women take advantage of this disposition of the law in order to get a living by wrongly accusing middle-class men of unlawful paternity (*The Annual Register*, 1834). In the midst of the class–gender war that was going on, some women might have tried to achieve a better life from a pension from a well-to-do gentleman. It is, however, difficult to know to what extent this happened and it seems unlikely to have been a very common practice. All things considered, the Commissioners, decided to suppress this disposition of the law which was more favourable to the unmarried mother and instead made *her* solely responsible for her child's upkeep. This enabled middle-class men to have access to lower-class women remorselessly and to exploit them – as a class – sexually as well as economically.

FROM THE NEW POOR LAW TO THE BEVERIDGE REPORT

The New Poor Law (NPL) of 1834 marked the end of paternalistic, local social relations as well as imposing a more efficient mode of domination on the lower classes. Although the only women it referred to were unmarried mothers and then in terms of punishment, it reinforced the sexual division of labour. The NPL intended to force the 'idle' to work, but it did not channel lower-class men and women into the same obligations; men had to enter production, women had to secure a man to depend on *before* they entered the reproductive sphere. The idle, able-bodied male pauper, like the single unsupported woman or worse, the unmarried mother, was subjected to the workhouse test. The women obviously fared worse than their male 'counterparts' in complying with what they were meant to do because there were twice as many women (and children) in workhouses as there were men. Nineteen per cent of all the female inmates were mothers with children, 50 per cent of all the children were of unknown fathers. This was true throughout the life of the workhouse system, which lasted until 1930 (Crowther, 1981). The Poor Law itself was only repealed in 1948. However, workhouses were still to be found as late as 1945 as the Curtis Report (Report of the Case of Children Committee, 1946) testifies.

The abolition, by the Bastardy Clauses of the New Poor Law, of the possibility of the unmarried mother receiving a pension from the father of her child caused riots among working-class women in the North of England (Rose, 1971). For the first time in recorded modern history, the women directly concerned became political actors and stood up collectively for their rights *as women*. In order to cool things down, the Commissioners re-established the possibility of getting an Affiliation Order, but the procedure was so complicated, and for such paltry results, that it was hardly ever used (Spensky, 1988).

Throughout the century, working-class women, who were under the moralising influence of upper-middle-class women philanthropists, came to judge unmarried motherhood through the eyes of the latter. As Roberts remarks, 'decades of Victorian attitudes had produced, at the turn of the twentieth century, a generation of working-class parents who were extremely prudish' (Roberts, 1984: 15). When *respectability* became the newly acquired wealth of the labouring classes, their attitude towards 'sexual deviance' hardened and no one remained to identify with unmarried mothers who were left to the Poor Law whenever they were considered 'undeserving' or to philanthropy whenever considered 'deserving'.

If the New Poor Law had been very much opposed by the classes it was meant to regulate, the Beveridge Report (1942), which was to embody all subsequent welfare laws, was supported by the working class as a whole. In the midst of the turmoil of the Second World War, the Beveridge Report redefined the terms of class as well as gender relations. Class relations were to be less violently exploitative thanks to the insurance system, which was to give dignity to the working man. On the other hand, women were redefined as dependent, even though when the Report was drafted, most of them were employed. As Smart has argued in relation to post-war family law: 'the government could be seen to be postponing any development in family law in an attempt to recreate a pre-war family structure' (Smart, 1984: 40). This is true of all the Acts that came out of the Beveridge Report. The only women the Poor Law had dealt with were unmarried mothers as they were seen to be the only ones to pose a problem; the women that interested Beveridge were married women and mothers, as they represented the ideal female model. For the first time an official document emphasised the importance of their *social* role, 'without which their husbands could not do their paid work and without which the nation could not continue' (Beveridge Report, 1942: 49, para. 107). No doubt, as Dale and Foster (1986) have argued, this must have been an important step for (married) women as the majority of them seem to have welcomed the new dispositions, even if a few feminist voices were heard against them. Not all feminists were against the Beveridge Report as the movement of what Banks (1981) called the 'Welfare Feminists', which had been strong in the inter-war period, was still alive. The Welfare Feminists, who influenced Beveridge through Eleanor Rathbone who had inspired him with the idea of children's allowances (Lewis, 1984; Lynes, 1984), had been asking for a public recognition of the social importance of women as wives and mothers for several decades. The fact that women were defined as ideally dependent, however, inevitably lead to a punishing attitude towards those who did not conform, especially unmarried mothers. While widows, who had not upset gender relations would get a pension *as of right* through the system of insurance and stay at home to raise their children, non-working unmarried mothers were granted a meagre means-tested allowance from the Assistance Board, which was very akin to the Poor Law that the new system was supposed to replace. While the non-working men who got a means-tested allowance had to prove that they had no work or savings, the women did too, but they also had to live in chastity, because if they were suspected of cohabiting with a man their allowance was withdrawn (National Council for the Unmarried Mother and her Child (NCUMC), 1968). Their sexuality was under constant scrutiny, unlike widows who were considered to have fulfiled the contract and were free to do what they would with their bodies. The philosophy of the Beveridge Report, which reflected the wide consensus of 'a conservative society described in the rhetoric of a radical ideology' (Wilson, 1980: 6), profoundly marked the social policies of the two decades following the Second World War.

THE RE-CONSTRUCTION OF CHILDHOOD AND MOTHERHOOD – MARRIED AND UNMARRIED – IN THE 1950s

Until the Second World War, unmarried motherhood had been considered as being the result of the seduction of an overcredulous girl, who was particularly weak in character, ignorant or mentally defective. Whenever an unmarried mother fell into the hands of a social worker, she was taught to be a 'good mother', that is, to provide for the material wellbeing of her child which included everything regarding its physical fitness. During the war, the impact of child psychology and, especially, child psychoanalysis was emphasised by the new interest in children caused by their massive evacuation to safe areas. This is a hypothesis which has not been thoroughly followed through but the fact is that, on the one hand, various general studies on children (Bowlby, 1940; Burlington and Freud, 1942) had child evacuees as their object and, on the other hand, the psychological suffering of these particular children caused psychologists to focus on this special group (Titmuss, 1950). The conclusion of most of the studies was that, in order to grow psychologically healthy, children should not be separated from their mothers. Not only was it bad for their own psychological development, since unhappiness can develop into neurosis if aggression is acted out against oneself, but it was even more dangerous if acted out against others as it might develop into delinquency. The Curtis Report (Report of the Case of Children Committee, 1946) emphasised the increase in delinquency during the war, 1941 being the peak year. Delinquency, according to a study of evacuated children by Bowlby, one of England's foremost child psychiatrists of the post-war period, 'can be traced to an early separation from the mother' (Bowlby, 1940: 190). Mothers were certainly more willing to accept these new theories than they might otherwise have been, because of the trauma of the children – and the guilt to the mothers – caused by the evacuations. In any case, the popularity of these theories which were widely publicised through women's magazines and the radio (Riley, 1983), restricted mothers' availability to work because, arising from the recognition of children's needs, their presence became a full-time requirement. This being the case, they had to stay at home.

This full-time availability of the mother – which meant that she depended on someone else for her subsistence – embodied in the Welfare Laws, brought the gaze of social work theory on the unmarried mother. Indeed, if the latter did not want to content herself with the bleak life of destitution available to her from subsistence on the meagre means-tested allowance provided by the new Welfare State, and if she did not want to deprive her child of a comfortable material environment, she would *have* to work and consequently her child would be deprived psychologically, or so it was thought.

The child's psychological wellbeing having become the main focus of attention, adoption was sometimes presented as the best solution available to unmarried mothers and was widely discussed after the war. In 1953, the National Association for Mental Health was asked to write a Memorandum on Adoption by the Home Office. The Association seemed to be perplexed by the double-bind implicitly contained in the new theories when applied to illegitimate children:

In principle, we may agree that the child's welfare should be given first place, but in practice this may open the way to difficult decisions. Should he be removed from a 'problem family' against the wish of his mother, and be adopted by wealthy and respectable citizens?

(National Association for Mental Health, 1953: 8)

It is made quite plain that unmarried mothers, who are neither wealthy nor respectable citizens, are to be included with the 'problem families'. The Association recommended that further study should be made on the adoption of *illegitimate children* because it did not have enough information. In the 1950s, new developments in social casework theories came from America which seemed to settle the question: being an unmarried mother was pathological. This was soon to be echoed by psychiatrists and journals of social work. Bowlby himself, who had always worked on child development, and never on female psychology, echoes these theories:

[I]t is the opinion of many social workers with psychiatric knowledge and experience of this problem that, with many girls, becoming an unmarried mother is neurotic and not just accidental. In other cases the girls are chronically maladjusted or defective.

(Bowlby, 1953: 3)

The most widely read book at the time on the subject was published in 1954 by Leontine Young, an American caseworker who specialised in work with unmarried mothers. Her book, *Out of Wedlock*, became a best seller among modern British social workers. It must be said that most social workers working on religious lines (the Moral Welfare workers) were very cautious about the psycho-analytically orientated interpretation of unmarried motherhood, as it negated the notion of free will without which there is no such thing as sin. They were torn between the wish to be modern and that of preserving a Christian interpretation of behaviour, but they gave in bit by bit towards the 1960s without ever surrendering completely (Spensky, 1988). Whilst psychoanalytically oriented social work had existed for more than 20 years in the United States, with no influence on British social work, it gradually gained a wide audience in Britain, partly because of the popularisation of psycho-analysis *vis à vis* evacuated children during the war and partly because of the growing cultural influence of the United States during and after the war. The post-war public was showered with what Kathleen Woodroofe called a 'psychiatric deluge' (Woodroofe, 1974: 118).

The pathologisation of unmarried motherhood was gradually constructed during the 1950s. It had started with the child needing a 'loving environment'. The mother would secure this environment, provided she depended on someone else for her material subsistence. Hence the healthy mother was one who was satisfied merely with *being* the healthy 'environment' for her child and having secured a husband *before* she had a baby. Consequently, the unmarried mother could not be very healthy.

Leontine Young's book was the first 'scientific' attempt to study the personality of unmarried mothers. Her theory was a break with those of the nineteenth century in that she asserted that the unmarried mother was the victim, 'not of a seducer, but of herself'. Unmarried motherhood was not, however, the result of careless sex, but rather of a plan carefully elaborated by the unconscious self: 'obviously, she wants a baby – but, specially an out-of-wedlock baby – without a husband' (Young, 1954: 28). It was this desire to bring into the world an illegitimate baby that *was* her pathology. Therefore, the fact that children were said to need the full-time care of their mother, added to the fact that unmarried motherhood was now considered to be a symptom of psychological unbalance, made social workers more inclined to think that the illegitimate child would be better off with 'a nice, married middle-class couple' than with a 'part-time, unbalanced single mother'. Even though Britain never used adoption as a mass remedy for illegitimacy, as only 25 per cent of British illegitimate children were ever adopted compared to 75 per cent of American ones (Pochin, 1969), it nevertheless filled the universe of social work discourse and greatly modified the practices of mother and baby homes.

HOMES FOR UNMARRIED MOTHERS AND THEIR CHILDREN AS REGULATORS OF SOCIAL RELATIONS: GENDER, CLASS AND 'RACE'

In order to be able to understand how dramatic the change of the homes in the 1950s was, a brief survey of how they functioned before the war is necessary.

Special homes for unmarried mothers and their illegitimate

offspring were opened by different missions towards the end of the nineteenth century.[1] They were created on the model of the penitentiary: the mother had to repent of her sin. She stayed in the home with her child for a year or two while she was taught a trade, usually that of domestic servant. When she came out, she was sent into service so that she could pay for the upkeep of her child who was sent to a foster mother. The natural mother was encouraged to visit her child as often as her job allowed her to. Only the mother of a first illegitimate child was considered as 'deserving' of a treatment better than that of the workhouse where other lone mothers were received, because there, she might be 'contaminated by tougher women', fail to repent and become a prostitute (*The Church of England Monthly Review*, 1858).

The homes were opened because of the increase of poor mothers wandering about or entering the workhouse with their illegitimate children, but they served also as a means of regulating women's sexuality and way of life. The woman who came out of the home was supposed to be very different from the one who had entered it: amended, 'respectable', employable and a 'good ' mother (i.e. one who provided for her child). The objective of the homes, which was to make unmarried mothers responsible towards their children and make sure they did not have a second one, remained almost unchanged (except for the length of stay which was reduced to 4 months in the inter-war period when domestic service ceased to be taught) until the aftermath of the Second World War when it metamorphosed dramatically because of the growing importance of child psychology and of psychoanalytically oriented social work.

In 1953, only one in five of all unmarried mothers ever entered a home (*Quarterly Review*, January 1955). This is only a minority but its impact on the discourse of social work on unmarried mothers, which was used as a disincentive for other young women to engage in pre-marital sex and risk a pregnancy, was more important. Those unmarried mothers who were cohabiting usually kept their child. Moreover, several studies undertaken in the 1950s and 1960s (Fielding, 1953; Gill, 1969; Methuven, 1948; Shaw, 1953) show that, if the parents of the young mother were willing to make a home for her and the child, the latter would not be abandoned; if not, then the chances were that adoption would be sought. Working-class parents seem to have been more willing to accept the situation than middle-class parents as the new inmates of the homes seemed to 'have come from a better background and are better educated than in pre-war days' ('Southwark', 1943 – see Archival Sources [1,2] p. 118).

Pre-war homes were considered by most unmarried mothers as a form of material help, essential whenever their parents would not or could not afford the financial burden of a new mouth to feed. During and after the war, working-class parents were better off than they would have been in pre-war time, thanks to full employment and welfare benefits. Middle-class parents (middle class is here taken in its wider meaning) on the other hand, were as conservative as they had been before and they refused to acknowledge the existence of their illegitimate grandchildren. More and more young middle-class mothers were to be found in the post-war homes. Most of them were there because they wanted to hide for a while or have their baby adopted. The ones who sought adoption were, according to the new theories, more mature and less pathological than those who kept their babies because the former had ambitions for themselves (Young, 1954). They were the ones who resembled their social worker most, as they belonged – or aspired to belong – to the same sort of social milieu where girls have enough psychological space to be allowed to have personal ambitions, either embodied in a university degree, a 'good' marriage or both. It was motherhood, however, which gave lower-class girls access to adulthood; why then – unless no one was ready to help them financially – would they get rid of the proof they had reached that stage, even though, ideally, they should have married beforehand?

Legitimised by Leontine Young's school of thought which theorised the different quality of mother-love according to the marital status of the mother, some matrons in mother-and-baby homes did not hesitate to put pressure on the mother so as to fulfil the desire of a middle-class-married-but-childless couple for a healthy baby. 'I have just the baby for you, but we shall have difficulty in getting her to part' says one in Kornitzer's study (1968). Young warned over-sensitive social workers against their own emotional reactions and against their belief that unmarried mothers felt as *they* would, if their children were removed. This was because, according to Young, unmarried mothers did not feel as attached to their offspring as other women did. This seemed to have been taken for granted by a number of social workers as shown by Kornitzer (1968). In 1951, the Church of England Moral Welfare Council had asked its workers not to put pressure on the unmarried mother in order to get her consent for adoption. In 1984, the National Council for One Parent Families issued a booklet on illegitimate children. A few letters by women who had abandoned their children in the 1950s and regretted it bitterly are published in it. One of them seems to summarise the others: 'At no stage was I consulted but I was made to feel so abjectly ashamed that I felt I could do nothing' (Derrick, 1986: 22). Obviously, not all mothers whose child was adopted consented under pressure but, whether it came from their parents or from a social worker, it was not uncommon. Curiously, when the psychological suffering of the child had become such a great concern, the psychological suffering of the young woman whose child was snatched from her – at a period when motherhood was so revered – was completely and 'scientifically' denied.

Thus, from the mid-1950s until the 1967 abortion legislation had time to have an effect in the 1970s, the home for unmarried mothers became a producer of legitimacy. The unmarried expectant mother would enter it a few weeks before confinement, then she would give birth, either in the home itself or in hospital and finally she would return to the home for a few weeks after which her baby would be adopted. The baby would be legitimised through adoption, the childless couple would acquire more legitimacy by having a child, and the mother would come out – apparently – as if nothing had happened, cured of her pathological unconscious urges. She would then be able to get married and, in her turn, bear legitimate children, this time, driven by more healthy, unconscious urges.

This production of legitimacy by the homes was new. In the past, they had been contented with preserving the legitimacy that already existed. The new function was added to the old one which it was still fulfiling. It was modified, however, by the impact of the war, which produced a new kind of 'client': the married woman. Towards the end of the conflict, as quite a considerable number of 'married mothers with children not their husbands'' applied ('Southwark', 1944), the homes were used partly to protect the threatened legitimacy of the returning soldiers' families and to maintain the husband's dominant position in its midst. This is quite clear in one of the reports to a particular home written by a social worker in 1944 who remarks proudly 'in some cases workers have been able to help towards a reconciliation between husband and wife and *where the husband so wished*, on the adoption of the child'. Those were the only married women who were catered for in the homes over this period. They were expected to be grateful to their husbands that they had not been thrown on to the street, but their possible feelings for their baby were considered as unimportant as those of the unmarried mothers quoted above.

Whenever the putative father of the illegitimate child was himself married, the homes protected his legitimate family by trying to preserve the married couple, because 'by making the girl independent of the man, they might help her to break with him, and so indirectly help the legitimate wife' (Report, November 1953); at least this is what was hoped. The family was thought to be in great danger of dissolution after the war, because of the numerous break-downs caused by lengthy separations. *Any* marriage was thought to be potentially good and social caseworkers helped, whenever needed by the newly created profession of sexologists, were there to make it work (Jeffreys, 1989). The mother-and-baby homes of this period form part of the variety of means used not only to preserve legitimacy, but also to produce it.

In most homes, the notion of what was not legitimate was even implicitly enlarged to include a possible 'improper' alliance across class, religious or ethnic barriers. Consequently, some women gave birth in the home, not because the putative father had run away or was married, but because marriage with a partner of the 'wrong' kind was socially unacceptable to both families. In the past, girls of the lower classes were already to be found in the homes because there was no question of them marrying the putative father whenever he was wealthier than they were. In the post-war era, some mothers belonged to the group considered superior and their parents opposed the marriage because it would bring shame on to the family and spoil the lineage. Legitimacy, taken in its legal sense in those cases, would have been considered socially illegitimate (i.e. unacceptable to most girls' parents and their social surroundings). This was the case with Joan who, 'aged 19, was admitted early because of difficult home circumstances, the father of the expected baby being West-African' (Report, December 1955). This was also the case with Mary whose boyfriend 'had gone back to

Nigeria, as both families were against mixed marriages' (Report, May 1956). Another putative father was Jewish while the mother was Church of England (Report, December 1953), another one was a turf accountant while the mother came from a 'respectable' family background (Report, December 1956). They were disqualified by the girl's family because they belonged to the 'wrong' ethnic, religious group or social class. Sometimes it was the putative father or his family who opposed the marriage for similar reasons. The babies born of these encounters were doubly illegitimate: as born outside wedlock and being born outside a socially acceptable milieu.

As there was a proliferation of adoptable babies, adoptive parents were able to be very 'choosy' as regards the quality of the child they wished to acquire. The homes, in conjunction with the redistribution of social status they performed, were able to provide prospective adoptive parents with 'good quality' babies. Those who did not reach parents' expectations were excluded from adoption. This happened to 'Kevin, aged three months [who had] been rejected for adoption as he might be albino' (Report, November 1955). Some adoptive parents even took the child back after a while whenever a flaw was discovered. Adoptive parents wanted a top-quality child and brought it back, even after they had looked after it for a few months, as if it was still under guarantee. This was the case of 'Bernard, aged six months', [who had] 'been returned by his adopters as he was found to be blind' (Report, December 1955). Eve's child would never be adopted as 'Eve, an assistant matron in a local authority school for retarded boys, has become pregnant by one of the pupils; here again, adoption will hardly be possible' (Report, October 1958).

Most of these children would have been kept by their parents had they been their own, but adoptive parents were more hard to please than natural parents. Some even complained about the educational level achieved by their adoptive child later in life as if this had come from nature and had nothing to do with nurture. In order to find a better match for the 'non academic child who proved to be such a disappointment to his University parents' (Shaw, 1953) social workers were asked to study the social background of the natural mother more thoroughly (it was as if they assumed that heredity was only passed through the mother). Everything was done to ensure that 'adopting parents get a better service from adoption societies (re risks) than ordinary parents do from nature' (Fielding, 1953). The range of choice was so wide that parents could order brothers and sisters for their first adoptee. Henry was one such child. He had been 'happily adopted and his father [had] written since to say he would like to adopt a brother for him' (Report, October 1955). Those children who were not accepted for adoption ended up with a foster mother if they were lucky or otherwise in a children's home, weighing even more heavily on their mother's guilt than the top-quality ones for whom comfortable homes were found.

Most adoptive parents not only wanted their adopted child to be healthy, but they also wanted it white and if possible from the same social class as themselves. Some even wanted it 'legitimate, if possible' (Edwards, 1949), but this might have been a bit too much to ask. The racial hostility faced by black, Asian and Oriental people in Britain is revealed quite bluntly by the reports of the urban homes. A drop of non-white blood made the adoption of this particular illegitimate child very unlikely. This was the case of Diana's baby, who could not be adopted 'as he [had] some Chinese blood' (Report, April 1958), Margaret's little girl was not adopted either, 'as her father [was] Indian' (Report, October 1958). In the 1960s this problem of illegitimate children of the 'wrong' ethnic kind increased because of the continuous flow of immigration of Caribbean workers which had started in the 1950s. It was not until the end of the 1960s though, that unmarried Caribbean mothers could be found in great numbers in the urban homes. During the 1960s, however, more white mothers entered them to give birth to a 'black' baby who was difficult to place because of its colour (Report, December 1962). White people's rejection was so strong that even foster mothers, who were paid to do the job, were reluctant to care for them. Those whose parents were both black were accepted with even more reluctance. Some foster mothers said they would take a coloured child 'if he [was] not too dark' (Antrobus, 1964: 39).

CONCLUSION

When Beveridge wrote his Report in 1942, the sexual division of labour had been upset by the need for women in war work. This affected gender relations which were less rigid than they had been in the past. The Report, however, reconstructed the traditional sexual division of labour and, consequently, froze gender relations in general in their pre-war state. This is the analysis made by one of the first feminist studies of this topic in the 1970s (Wilson, 1977) and it remains a persuasive argument. More recently Dale and Foster (1986) have added to the previous analysis that this return to 'normal' must have been acceptable to most women because even though 'the Beveridge Report excited angry reaction from many feminists . . . most feminists welcomed the post-war reforms as improving women's material position and status in society' (Dale and Foster, 1986: 3, 17).[2] The fact is that it gave housewives a legal status while legalising their dependence on men.

More recently, Smart has argued that it was the agitation raised by the Family Endowment Society led by Eleanor Rathbone which helped married women more than the Report as such, since it succeeded in giving mothers direct access to the family allowance rather than their husbands (Clarke et al., 1987). This certainly was very important for married mothers because, on the one hand, it pointed to the fact that 'the family wage did not automatically go towards the support of the dependent members of the family' and on the other hand that 'the acceptance of the proposal that married women should be entitled to receive benefit direct from the state provided a major plank in the argument that women should not be forced to look to men for their, and their children's economic survival' (Clarke et al., 1987: 109). Unmarried mothers, however, seldom had more than one child and were, consequently, not entitled to child allowance at this time. Moreover, the money they were able to get from the state when they were not in the labour market was means tested and not part of the contributions based insurance system celebrated by the Report.

The dominant discourse in the 1950s and 1960s of the contented housewife and mother of happy children, nourished by the legal, medical and social-work professions, consequently constructed unmarried mothers as no more than social deviants who, as such, were not to be consulted. This idea of 'deviancy' was constructed in scientific terms by the new theories developed by psycho-analytically orientated social work which stated that women who bore children without a husband were pathological. This rapidly led to thinking that the adoption of their children would be the best solution for both mother and child.

My analysis of the reports from homes for unmarried mothers

reflects this treatment of the female social deviant and of that of her offspring. Through the use of adoption, not only did the homes reduce the figures of illegitimacy as infant mortality had done in the past but, at the same time, it also produced legitimacy. The home acted like a sorting-out centre, which redistributed statuses. First of all, it gave a legal status to the illegitimate child through adoption, legitimising at the same time a childless marriage and then allowing the unmarried mother to marry and thus to produce legitimate children. Moreover, it allowed her to get rid of the fruits of a relationship with a man of the 'wrong' social group, namely the 'wrong' religion, the 'wrong' social class or the 'wrong' ethnic group. The unmarried mother who did not wish to furnish the home with someone else's legitimate child avoided it whenever she could. On an ideological level the new welfare state had marginalised unmarried mothers, possibly more than the Poor Law had done, by setting up two different systems of redistribution of wealth of which one, based on the insurance principle, was dignified while the other, based on assistance, was not. Unless they were in the labour market and had access to child-care facilities, unmarried mothers either accepted the undignified means-tested assistance in order to keep their child, or went into a home which organised adoption for them. They were making shift with the only options that were open to them. Both could, with some reason, be regarded as punitive.

NOTES

1 The first two homes specialising in residential work with unmarried mothers and their children were founded in 1860 by the Female Mission. More homes were founded by different missions during the last quarter of the century.

2 There must have been some sort of collective unconscious resistance, however, because the number of women in the labour market increased by 17.4 per cent (51.6 per cent for married women) between 1950 and 1963 (Klein quoted by Smart, 1984: 53). It does not mean though that married women did not think their primary duty was that of mother, as a large number of them were part-timers and mothers of children under school-age seldom worked. The State ignored – and still does – the problems of the working mother and child care which was organised on a private basis.

ARCHIVAL SOURCES

1 Yearly Reports (1895–1968) of Moral Welfare, the former name of Wel Care. This association, which was created in 1895 under the name of 'Diocesan Association for the Care of Friendless Girls' was to become 'Wel Care' in 1961. It is sometimes referred to as 'Rochester' or 'Southwark' as it corresponds to the part of London, south of the river, which I have studied more thoroughly. Moral Welfare provided Britain with most of its homes for unmarried mothers. It also had a counselling service.

2 The monthly reports (1904 – 1968) of a home for unmarried mothers created in 1903 which I refer to as Reports refer to a particular home in the text. The names of the people involved have been changed as they are still alive and have a right to privacy. These reports were in manuscript form and had never been consulted before.

Chapter 6

Representing childhood
The multiple fathers of the Dionne quintuplets
Mariana Valverde

The historical emergence of 'neglected children', 'unfit mothers' and other identities found in the toolkits of social welfare officials has been amply documented in recent historical critiques of the apparent naturalness of psychological and social-work labels (Garland, 1985; Gordon, 1989). By now most critical scholars regard the taxonomies of social welfare not as descriptive classifications of naturally occurring species but rather as ideologically constructed conceptual systems whose historical origins and political function can be unearthed. We are beginning to see that 'the neglected child', for instance, is not an empirical fact but a category of social work. Nevertheless we still want to believe that as labels for specific behaviours change over time, there is still something out there called 'child welfare', or, at the very least, there are still such entities as 'children'. Now, just as Riley (1988) has recently argued that what is or is not a woman is determined in historically specific ways through shifts in discourses, so too it is possible to argue that the category 'children' (as occurring in social work and other dominant practices/discourses) is only contingently related to human physiology: what is or is not a matter for child welfare is not *a priori* obvious, as the present case study shows. Rather than follow the usual social historians' practice of documenting the emergence of a new identity, however, this study shows the category of childhood disappearing. In the golden age of North American childrearing experts (Arnup, 1990), a set of quintuplets born in rural Ontario in 1934 were constructed by various agencies as models or representations of childhood, but not as children. The Dionne sisters, I will argue, were no more 'children' (for purposes of the guardianship disputes) than Mickey Mouse is a mouse.

Elzire Dionne, a French-speaking farm woman who already had

five children, gave birth to five identical girls in May of 1934. The doctor did not believe that the tiny babies would live, and most probably neither did the parents. Oliva Dionne, their father, signed a contract with Chicago fair promoters promising to let the girls be exhibited if and when they were healthy. Denouncing this contract, the Ontario provincial government (which under the Canadian constitution has responsibility for child welfare and other social services) obtained a judicial order taking the children away from their parents' custody and control. The government had a shiny new hospital built across the road from the farm, and soon proceeded to draw tourists to this hitherto remote spot by exhibiting the girls through one-way glass to hundreds of thousands of tourists from all over North America. As time went on, a great deal of money accumulated in the girls' trust fund, as companies bought the right to use references to the famous prodigies of science/nature in order to sell products from condensed milk to typewriters. After many years of challenging the English-speaking doctor directly and the government indirectly, the girls' father was eventually able to regain custody over the girls, as the Francophone community of Ontario and the Catholic church mobilised to defend one of their own against the interfering Anglo-Protestant government. The girls, however, disliked their biological parents and had nothing in common with their other siblings. They were emphatically not happy ever after.

When I began to research the 'case' of the Canadian Depression starlets, and more particularly to document the guardianship process, I thought of my work as dealing with the regulation of children and motherhood in the context of an emerging welfare state. The province of Ontario, the largest and richest in Canada, was the pioneer in social services and other branches of welfare, and so I hoped that work on this case would shed light on larger processes of state formation and family regulation throughout English Canada. It was thus surprising to note that the popular phrase of the 1920s and after, 'child welfare', did not occur anywhere in the twelve boxes of government pap rs concerning the guardianship.[1] Press clippings invariably showed public officials zealous to defend the welfare of the girls no matter what the cost to the public purse, but when speaking among themselves, the guardians, male politicians and administrators never used the language of child welfare. They spoke only about two things: the monetary value, especially in tourist revenues, that the quintuplets represented, and the possible electoral value of the Liberal Government's image as a paternal state.

Saved from certain infant death by the miracles of modern science but reared in the bracing air of northern backwoods, and provided with a 'non-degenerate' genetic background as well as with every environmental advantage, the quintuplets were the paradigm of 1930s childhood.[2] But, just as Plato argued long ago that it is a category confusion to think that the idea of beauty is itself beautiful, so too, this paradigm of childhood, the set of five undistinguishable smiling faces, was a creation of discourse, a cultural institution, more than a group of 'real' children. Perhaps if they had grown up as Annette, Cecile, Yvonne, Marie and Emilie they might have become children. As it was, they acquired a social identity only as a *sui generis* unique product – the Quintuplets, with the word capitalised and made into a trademark.

The government's handling of the guardianship shows that kinship and household forms, parenting, maternity and paternity are not always directly regulated as such by a specialised part of the state. On the contrary, they are subject to much indirect regulation emanating from unlikely sites within and without the state. It has been pointed out that tax law, for instance, acts in such a way as to regulate marriage and family practices (Lewis, 1983; Resources for Feminist Research, 1988). The present study shows that the Dionne family had their internal organisation as well as their external relations shaped not only by the government's takeover of the babies but also by the myriad commercial contracts fostered by the guardians. For example, photographs of the quintuplets taken from 1935 to 1944 never showed the parents. Although this exclusion helped to legitimise the government's stigmatisation of Mr and Mrs Dionne as unfit parents, the more immediate reason for it was that the contract for exclusive rights of quints' photographs did not extend to pictures of their parents and siblings. The contracts thus regulated family life, but not qua family, and not via the social welfare apparatus. Having one's kin networks organised by trademark law and commercial contracts is rather different from being subjected to child protection agents. In general, indirect social regulation is different from the direct regulation exerted by specialised agencies upon their targets, and hence requires innovative research methods (see Valverde, 1990; 1991).

From the official standpoint, the Dionne quintuplets figured as capital, mainly tourist-industry capital. The names Annette, Cecile, Yvonne, Emilie and Marie hardly ever appear in the government papers, with the interesting and not accidental exception of income tax forms.[3] Given the blatant commercial exploitation of these five children, it is tempting to denounce the government in the same language employed by the dozens of mothers who wrote to the Premier to protest (or in some cases to conditionally approve) the government's actions. Many of these letters question whether the Dionne sisters' scientific and cultural uniqueness warranted the extraordinary arrangements made for them, and deploy concepts such as 'normal childhood'.[4] Humanist conceptions of innocent and properly individualised childhood are (and were) the obvious alternative to the government's position. But moral condemnations of child exploitation do little but uncritically legitimise 'modern' childrearing perspectives (Sutherland, 1976). What if the girls had been handled by a benevolent agency? Or even by their own mother? What if they had indeed been treated as 'children'? Did their siblings and other contemporaries live happy childhoods? If all social relations tend to elicit familiar narratives with recognisable modes of closure, little children as a social construct surely elicit the most powerful narratives: but our desire to deliver the quintuplets from evil kings need not lead to perpetuating the myth that normal families contain happy children.

THE EVOLUTION OF THE GUARDIANSHIP

Dr Allan Roy Dafoe, the Anglophone doctor who assisted two Francophone midwives at the quintuplets' birth on 28 May 1934, intimated to the girls' father that his children would not live. Ranging in weight from $1\frac{1}{2}$–$2\frac{1}{2}$ lb, the babies were visibly fragile. Incubators were not to be found anywhere in the neighbourhood, and in any case the farmhouse did not have electricity. While the babies and their mother struggled on the brink of death, the father, Oliva Dionne, appears to have been primarily concerned about his financial responsibility. When approached by a Chicago fair exhibit promoter interested in the quintuplets, Oliva Dionne consulted his parish priest. The priest apparently gave his blessing to the Chicago offer, as did Dr Dafoe, who was quite sure the girls' failing health would prevent their removal to Chicago (the contract specified that the girls would not be moved contrary to medical advice) (Berton, 1977; Nimey, 1986). Neither the priest nor the doctor, however, incurred the government's wrath. Choosing its target carefully, the newly elected Liberal Attorney General gathered the news media and painted a sinister portrait of the girls' father as a greedy and ignorant peasant who offered no resistance to the siren-song of American commercialism.[5]

The respectable Toronto daily the *Globe* stated: 'Acting in his function as "parens patriae" – father of the people – [Attorney General] Mr Roebuck has obtained, through a North Bay solicitor, a judicial order appointing guardians for the quintuplets, and so defeated the "perfidious contract" ' between the Chicago promoters and Oliva Dionne.[6] Roebuck posed as the knight protecting the nation's honour, saying: 'If exploiters from American cities come to Canada to pull off this sort of racket, they need not expect the Attorney General's office or the courts to stand idly by.'[7]

Successfully appealing to the popular image of Canada as a pure maiden needing defence from the lustful Uncle Sam, the government named four guardians, all male, and, almost as important, all Liberals (including Dr Dafoe and the girls' grandfather, Olivier Dionne). Whatever records were kept of the deliberations of the first guardianship have disappeared; it is nevertheless clear that Dr Dafoe behaved as the only guardian, engaging in commercial contracts involving the quintuplets as well as himself. As scientists and doctors around the world expressed amazement that the girls were still alive (no other quintuplets had lived beyond a few weeks), Dr Dafoe was hailed as a hero combining the wisdom of urban science with the natural common sense of a country doctor. Dr Dafoe, who was in fact not much of a scientist and acted on daily instructions from his obstetrician brother in Toronto, promoted the physical separation of the quintuplets from their family, with the backing of the government. A nursery was quickly built across the road from the Dionne farm and significantly named 'the Dafoe Hospital'. Dr Dafoe managed both the hospital and the girls, with the actual labour provided by a succession of nurses. Nurse De Kiriline, who was firmly in charge for the first few months, later admitted that she had treated the parents and siblings as nothing but unhygienic nuisances (Berton, 1977: 71–3).

The hospital featured modern appliances in a sterilised environment, but it simultaneously represented rustic Canada through its log-cabin exterior. It was built mostly through public donations and Red Cross funds;[8] but the government, in the first of many moves to appear as a bountiful father, claimed that it had spent $20,000 on the hospital, and that more money could not possibly be spent on the rest of the family.[9]

In March of 1935, when it had become apparent that the girls would probably live to be adults, the government sought to replace the judicial order by a more permanent guardianship agreement. A special law was drawn up making the girls wards of the Crown,[10] with the Crown's authority being exercised by the provincial minister of welfare, David Croll. Croll headed a board of guardians whose main members were Dr Dafoe and, in a policy reversal, the quints' father, Oliva Dionne, who had already begun to stir up Francophone interests against the government. During the debate in the provincial legislature on this bill, the government revealed its intentions: 'The government is also considering improvements to the Dafoe hospital that may include a large glass-covered solarium where tourists and visitors would be able to see the quintuplets.'[11] The opposition Conservatives never thought to point out that the government was about to repeat the action of the 'greedy' father.[12] It also failed to raise questions about a further curious statement by Croll, namely that the money already accumulating in the trust fund might be invested not in a regular stock portfolio but in Government of Ontario bonds.[13] Through these two admissions the government was frankly revealing its intentions to use the quintuplets to boost the province's financial position. But the lie about the tax money supposedly spent on the hospital, coupled with the general ignorance of the fact that the doctor, the business manager, the nurses and even the provincial policemen on duty at the hospital were all paid out of the trust fund and were not on the government payroll, created the impression that the province was spending money protecting the girls. This may have been reassuring to parents trying to cope with Depression unemployment and low wages while reading in the papers that relief officers were pushing sterilisation and birth control on to poor parents.[14] As the opposition rose to ask if the province was being reimbursed for its expenditures, Croll again misled the voters about the direction in which the dollars flowed: 'We regard what the province has done as a whole-hearted contribution from all the people of the Province.'[15]

A few hours before the quintuplets Bill received royal assent, huge headlines in Toronto papers announced that the government had cleverly foiled a kidnap attempt by unnamed American commercial interests. Croll refused to give details about this convenient threat (undocumented in the provincial police files),[16] and an anonymous government official once more projected the government's greed onto others, declaring: 'Once beyond the King's guardianship, the quintuplets are a potential gold mine.'[17]

Given the rather distant relationship of the Ontario Government to the British Crown, the frequent use by government officials of the name and image of the King indicates an attempt to deploy the image of autocratic but benevolent political fatherhood to legitimise the actions of a lacklustre and highly partisan sub-national government. The law also made the girls instant princesses, symbolically if not legally. 'These children are our own royal family', Croll proudly declared (Berton, 1977:132). The twice-daily showings of the quintuplets in their playground to tourists jamming the 1,000-car parking lot could thus be implicitly justified without fear of commercial taint. Princesses, after all, have a duty to appear before their loyal subjects regardless of personal inconvenience or threat to their privacy.

The discourse of royalty furthermore legitimised the girls' complete segregation from other children, and for that matter from their parents and other siblings (who were not royal). The whole essence of royalty is separation from commoners, and loneliness is its unfortunate but inevitable price. While numbers of commoner girls around Ontario were made wards of the Children's Aid Society, the quintuplets were portrayed more as princesses shut in their castle than as wards of the state.[18]

The princess rhetoric was a very effective alternative to the freak-shows commercialism which had irreparably tainted the parents' public image and which the government was at pains to avoid, in its rhetoric if not in its actions.[19] By the 1930s, live exhibitions of Siamese twins and the like were deemed incompatible with twentieth-century notions of innocent childhood. Public display of children now assumed a mediated form, most notably in Hollywood musicals featuring Shirley Temple. The modernity of cinematic display haunted the Dionne sisters in later years, as we shall see, but initially official rhetoric, even when presented on newsreels, was reminiscent of old-fashioned fairy tales.

As in fairy tales about kings with three pretty daughters, the presence of a royal father in the Dionne story served to draw attention away from the girls' legal and factual motherlessness. Although the father was now included on the board (even if he was outnumbered), the mother was totally excluded. Croll said that 'when the Bill was being drafted it was suggested that Mrs Dionne be named a guardian, but the lawyer [whose lawyer is not clear] pointed out it might involve journeys which Mrs Dionne might not be prepared to take and it was thought that naming the father would be sufficient.'[20] As a matter of fact, Elzire Dionne travelled to the nearby city in which guardianship meetings were held, North Bay, 2 weeks after Croll's statement, to address a meeting of the Federation des Femmes Canadiennes Francaises. Not believing that it was sufficient to 'name the Father', she announced she was 'anxious the board of guardians include herself and two other women, both mothers, who could understand her longing to be with the babies as much as possible.'[21] The mother's call for gender parity on the board went unheeded, however. Later on the press would give sympathetic portraits of Mrs Dionne as wronged mother, but in the early days she was portrayed as illiterate (because she did not speak English) and as a lazy overeater (she did weigh about 200 pounds, unfortunately for her public image) and hence as no fit mother to princesses, even if her qualifications to care for her other five children were unchallenged.

In early 1937, a new epoch in the guardianship began as Croll gave his place on the Board of Guardians to the province's Official Guardian, Percy D. Wilson, a Liberal lawyer. From the careful records kept by Wilson, it appears that he saw his role as a dual one: first, preserving the public image of the government as a 'good father' to the quintuplets, and second, mediating between Dr Dafoe and Oliva Dionne, whose mutual hostility had by no means decreased. The benevolent patriarch image required that contracts be scrutinised for possible ideological flaws: some products were deemed to be unsuitable to associate with the quintuplets' picture, and all manufacturers granted licences had to meet Wilson's standards for dignified publicity. Making a full report to Premier Hepburn shortly after taking over from Croll, Wilson said nothing about the welfare of the children, emphasising only the need to promote and sell the quintuplets, if only to pay the skyrocketing legal fees.[22]

On Wilson's recommendation, a full-time business manager for the guardianship was appointed: Keith Munro, a reporter with a keen eye for business (who would later capitalise on his quint management experience by setting up a public-relations firm in New York's Madison Avenue). Munro was paid a salary of $500 a month out of the trust fund, five times more than the parents. Munro and Wilson made frequent trips to New York to meet with business contacts and lawyers, and the two men developed a very close friendship through their work on the guardianship's finances.[23] This work was by no means philanthropic child protection: Wilson charged every plate of fish and chips eaten in North Bay hotels to the quints' trust fund, not his own government department, and towards the end of the guardianship he even collected payments of $800 per year for the regular administration of the fund (on top of his salary).[24]

Also in early 1937, the provincial government sought to protect the valuable name and image of the quintuplets through a special trademark law, which had to be passed by the federal government since the province had no jurisdiction over trademarks. This badly drafted law, not in keeping with the provisions of the general trade-mark law, had more of a symbolic than a coercive effect. Two lengthy opinions from expensive lawyers concurred that the law would not stand judicial scrutiny, but that it nevertheless helped to create the impression that nobody could use the word 'quintuplets' without paying royalties to the guardianship. New York lawyer Arthur Garfield Hays put it starkly:

> The obtaining of some trade-marks, the licensing of the names and the reputation of the Quintuplets has resulted in a general public belief that these terms should be regarded as a monopoly. Business men hesitate to infringe when threatened with a law suit. We have on occasion been hard put to it to lay a foundation for legal rights when we have been squarely faced with the question, but we have not yet failed in persuading any such user to cease his unfair use. The argument that a a law suit for infringement would publicize the user as one who is attempting to take money from babies, has usually been effective as a deterrent.
>
> (A.G. Hays to P.D. Wilson, 28 Jan. 1938,
> 'Trade Mark' file, Box 9, DQG)

From 1937 until 1940, the guardians' monthly meetings in North Bay drew together Dafoe, Oliva Dionne, Munro, Wilson (most of the time) and Judge J.A. Valin, appointed as guardian because of his relatively neutral role as an English-educated francophone.[25] In December 1939 Wilson, although impatient with Oliva Dionne's constant stonewalling, supported his demand to have Dr Dafoe removed from the Board. Dafoe remained as the quints' doctor, however, and during 1940 and 1941 the quints' health was used as the football in a match fought bitterly by Dr Dafoe against Oliva Dionne, with Wilson as the referee. The children's education was also the object of bitter disputes and was thus constantly interrupted. Wilson's exasperation grew to the point that he advised that Anglophone teachers be replaced by French-speaking nuns, since 'the parents would, perhaps, be more amenable to their authority, or at least more amenable to them than any other authority.'[26]

With public opinion increasingly siding with the parents and calling for unification of the two Dionne families, Wilson advised his superiors that the government would eventually have to hand the quintuplets to their father. Apart from feeling harassed by Oliva Dionne, Wilson also feared the groundswell of French Canadian opinion, which was increasingly connecting the girls' education and upbringing to their centuries-old cause. (The right of Francophone parents to send their children to Francophone schools was then, as it still is now, one of the main rallying cries of French Canadians outside Quebec.) Wilson wrote: 'The reunion should clear away any chance that the children might be used, even in a small way, as an instrument to break down English speaking and French speaking relations.'[27]

The ante was upped in 1941 by the Catholic church. An article portraying the Dionnes as a good Catholic family divided by an uncaring government was published in the US Catholic magazine *America* and partly reprinted in a Toronto Catholic newspaper. A couple of months later, American journalist Lillian Barker wrote scornfully that the Government of Ontario could not have foreseen 'that such human mites would soon become a human gold mine to their Province.'[28]

The combined efforts of Anglophone Catholics, Francophones, and Dionne himself succeeded in obtaining a government promise to unite the two families. High-level meetings involving several cabinet ministers were held to discuss the location of the new home/homes and the children's educational programme. In the end, the Minister of Public Works ordered the building of a new home for all of the Dionnes, and Wilson declared he would not oppose family reunification as long as the children were still exhibited in public 'by way of attracting tourists to the province.'[29] The transfer of custody took several years to be implemented. On their tenth birthday the quintuplets were sent to live with their parents and siblings. The 'happy reunion' trumpeted in the press was merely apparent, however.[30] The girls hated doing farm chores, were virtual strangers to their siblings and did not like either parent very much. Their experience of a miserable adolescence is beyond the scope of this essay, but it is curious that their own published account has not managed to destroy the still-prevailing popular picture of a simple, rustic family reunited after many trials (Brough, 1965).

MAXIMISING THE VALUE OF A STATE RESOURCE

Although drained by legal fees of several thousand dollars per year, the regular wages of about twenty people, and the unlimited expenses of the guardians, the quintuplets' trust fund managed to accumulate about half a million dollars by 1 April 1937 and over $850,000 by January 1940.[31] In 1941 Judge Valin told the press that 'the babies are now worth a million dollars' and freely admitted that 'most of their money is invested in Ontario government bonds.'[32]

Boosting the province's credit by the assured large-scale purchase of bonds was nevertheless secondary to the main function of the quintuplets as a tourist attraction. The Quintland complex, complete with large souvenir shops run by Oliva Dionne and by the ex-midwives, was a Mecca for vacationing families enjoying the relatively new pastime of automobile tourism. By 1936, Quintland equalled Niagara Falls as Canada's leading tourist attraction. It furthermore provided a great deal more of indirect revenue because, while the Falls are right on the border, Americans had to travel for at least three days within Ontario on their baby-gazing pilgrimage, spending money all along. The road was paved and there were plenty of bathrooms, but the site exuded rustic charm. The government was well aware of the need to maximise the 'wilderness' character of Quintland (while of course providing physical comforts to the motoring Americans); when a new site was being planned for the new reunited family, the Attorney General 'emphasized that the site chosen should be picturesque, healthy, with a supply of good water. He urged that the site be one which could be regarded as typically Northern Ontario.'[33]

Like Lake Nipissing and the Canadian Shield, the Dionne girls were presumed to be naturally destined to be a sight for the tourist gaze. But unlike the granite shield, the girls were also expected to emulate the artifice of Shirley Temple and perform (Eckert, 1987). While as babies their picture had sufficed to sell calendars and milk products, by the time they were 3 or 4 they were expected to make radio appearances. Making their collective voice into a commodity proved rather difficult, partly because they lacked Shirley Temple's enterprising mother/manager and partly because their native tongue was French. Teaching the quintuplets English was, in the eyes of the guardians, the key that would open Hollywood's doors and ensure that the quintuplets' value would not fall as they lost their baby cuteness. Munro, haunted by the spectre of declining revenues, warned Wilson that Twentieth-Century Fox's lucrative contract would not be renewed unless the girls' human capital was increased through teaching them not only English but American-like behaviour:

> I am firmly convinced that a great deal depends on this next picture as far as the Quintuplets themselves are concerned. If they appear in a picture and are unable to speak English and behave as people of the United States think four-year-old children should behave, . . . the public would lose interest in the children to an extent that would endanger their earning capacity.
>
> (Munro to Wilson, 18 January 1938,
> 'Twentieth-Century Fox' file, Box 9, DQG)

It is probable that the daily squabbles in the nursery were not conducive to teaching the quintuplets anything; in any case, for whatever reason, 2 years later the girls still did not speak English. Munro highlighted the 'loss of revenue' that was already happening due to this failure to invest, and, for once acting in concert, Dr Dafoe and Oliva Dionne agreed to write the government to request an English teacher.[34]

The girls did learn some English, but, perhaps sensing that English might further estrange them from their parents, did not necessarily speak it on command. In a fiasco that rocked both the American media establishment and the provincial government, the quintuplets, scheduled to make a 'tasteful' live appearance on the American radio nework CBS, suddenly refused to speak English. While a producer vainly struggled to elicit words from the girls, Yvonne reportedly said to a nurse (in French), 'I don't want to speak English', and her sisters stood in silent solidarity with her.[35] Their act of resistance, denounced by hundreds of angry letters to Ontario's tourist bureau, was probably related to the fact that the girls had also been scheduled to sing the popular wartime song 'There'll Always Be An England'. A couple of months earlier Munro had already heard rumours that the girls were being told (by unnamed but obviously Francophone adults) not to sing in English and to especially avoid 'There'll Always Be An England.'[36]

While making the girls speak English and act American was the main means contemplated by the guardians to increase the value of their product, the smallest detail of the girls' lives could become the object of revenue-maximising projects. One example perhaps suffices to illustrate this: the 'Hair' file kept by the Official Guardian. Documents and photographs in this file tell a story of constant struggles between Mrs Dionne, who thought the girls' hair was fine as nature had made it, and the business manager and the Official Guardian, who both insisted that the girls' hair required the attentions of world-class experts. After a request by American photo syndicates, Munro wrote several letters to Wilson demanding 'an expert hairdresser'. He supported his claim with a packet of 8 x 10 photographs showing the girls with long, slightly wavy hair, described as 'ugly' in the accompanying letter.[37] The media quickly publicised this controversy, reporting that Mrs Dionne 'has forbidden Munro to bring world- famous hairdressers and fashion designers to the Dafoe Hospital'. The conclusion drawn was that Elzire Dionne 'opposes all efforts to modernize the little girls.'[38]

Elzire Dionne's claim over the physical appearance of the girls was thus questioned not because she was an unfit mother but because she opposed the combined forces of modernity and capital maximisation. Child welfare was not in question; what was at stake was the value of a resource which, although in some ways 'natural', needed constant cultural upgrading. As the 1940s wore on, the issue of 'modernising' the girls became more pressing, since the war and the girls' loss of baby cuteness threatened to dry up the income. Showing an anxiety over finances that he never showed about the girls' wellbeing, Wilson warned Munro:

> It must ever be kept in mind, in view of the general conditions, of the possibility of the earning power of the Quintuplets falling below their necessary expenditures. In other words, the time will come when the capital will have to be temporarily drawn upon for their maintenance.
>
> (Wilson to Munro, 19 January 1942, 'Paramount' file, Box 8, DQG)

As early as 1941, a former executive of the US entertainment giant Pathé News had reported to Munro that 'everybody in the picture business, with the exception of myself, seems to feel that the Quintuplets are dead.'[39] If the quintuplets' value had continued to rise exponentially, it is unlikely that the government would have willingly relinquished custody to the father. But with the quintuplets being pronounced media-dead, it was perhaps easy for Wilson and the government to lose some power and some revenue while posing as a white knight returning the girls to their ancestral home. The fact that it was the same knight who had stolen them in the first place was, tactfully, not brought up by the media.

CONTESTING STATE OWNERSHIP

Thus far it has been shown that the five Dionne girls were a valuable resource whose ownership was contested by the state, Dr Dafoe, the father, and the Francophone and Catholic communities, though the latter did not seek direct ownership but rather supported the father, who in turn supported the Francophone Catholic education system. These were not the only players in the bizarre game of paternal Monopoly, however; the new science of child psychology and the mass media also sought to define, and to some extent to own, the girls.

The new science of child psychology had its main Canadian promoter in Dr William Blatz, founder of the Institute for Child Study at the University of Toronto. Blatz rejected both traditional common-sense parenting and the eugenic beliefs prevalent in the

1920s, and declared that a good environment and scientific discipline were the two keys to healthy childhood. He believed that parents generally were far too emotional to be good child-rearers: both anger and affection were thus banned (in theory at least) from Blatz's model nursery. No physical punishment, no shouting, no sudden expressions of love were allowed. The children were literally enveloped in a minute-by-minute unvarying routine, and if they departed from the routine, their punishment was to be sent to a room by themselves until their emotions had disappeared.

Although Blatz was a leader of the 'progressive' wing of the child-study movement, a profoundly blind belief in modernity and in bureaucratic (rather than personal) discipline suffuses all his work (Dehli, 1990; Strong-Boag, 1988: 165–6). A couple of passages from Blatz's popular book on the Dionne girls are revealing:

A parent's love without understanding cannot compensate for ignorance.

A scheme of discipline may then be defined as a plan under which a child may best learn to fit into the civilisation in which he lives. . . . There is no question of obedience or disobedience, or of non-conformity. These problems arise only where the educator lacks confidence in himself or his civilisation.

(Blatz, 1938: 128–9)

While the children attending Blatz's nursery school went home at five, the Dionnes were under 24-hour surveillance by Blatz's female workers between 1935 and 1938. A slew of scientific papers were produced from the thousands of measurements taken of the girls' bodies and minds. The accompanying charts, reproduced from one of the studies, speak volumes about the scientists' world-view, while giving little or no information about the girls themselves (Figs 7.1 and 7.2).

These studies were rather trivial: the quints were found to be indeed identical, and their intellectual and emotional development was found to be slow for their age, not suprising given their low birth weight and unstimulating environment. But they furthered the individual careers of psychologists and scientists as well as the public image of behaviourist psychology, then in its infancy (Blatz et al., 1937; McArthur and Ford, 1937).

There is no record of opposition by the Dionne parents to Blatz's educational philosophy. In fact, there are some suggestions that

Figure 7.1

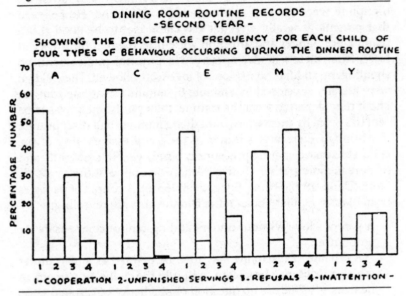

DINING ROOM ROUTINE RECORDS
-SECOND YEAR-

SHOWING THE PERCENTAGE FREQUENCY FOR EACH CHILD OF
FOUR TYPES OF BEHAVIOUR OCCURRING DURING THE DINNER ROUTINE

1-COOPERATION 2-UNFINISHED SERVINGS 3-REFUSALS 4-INATTENTION -

Source: MacArthur and Ford (1937)

Elzire Dionne, contrary to her press image as a backward peasant, held some admiration for modern education methods. A report by an ally of Elzire's, the French Vice-president of the Ontario Liberal Women's Association, held that Mrs Dionne wanted the 'intelligent culture' and 'scientific training' provided to the quintuplets extended to her other children. Mrs Dionne reportedly believed that the quintuplets' superior education might even 'make for an inferiority complex on the part of her other children'. Even though Mrs Dionne (or her ally) was tranparently using the discourse of scientific psychology to support her demand that the government build a special school for all her kids, it may be that she was not impervious to the aura of scientific childrearing, and derived some pride from 'the Quints being models for Canadian parents to follow in raising their families.'[40]

Whatever the prestige of science in the eyes of the mother and/or the father, the fact remained that Dr Blatz and his workers were Anglophones from Toronto in alliance with Dr Dafoe, so they became targets of Oliva Dionne's anger. In February of 1938 Oliva

Figure 7.2

Child	Routines	A Frequency of non-compliance for each child 16 days			B Frequency of authoritative measures 48 days		
		1st Half	2nd Half	Total Period	1st Half	2nd Half	Total Period
Annette	Sleep	18	11	29	4	1	5
	Dressing	13	16	29	4	3	7
	Washing	10	8	18	0	1	1
	Toilet	28	11	39	4	2	6
	Eating	33	18	51	14	5	19
	Play–Indoor	38	33	71	10	5	15
	Outdoor	36	6	42	1	4	5
	Unusual Situations	2	3	5	0	0	0
	Totals	178	106	284	37	21	58
Cecile	Sleep	11	9	20	4	5	9
	Dressing	10	14	24	4	2	6
	Washing	14	5	19	3	0	3
	Toilet	18	14	32	9	1	10
	Eating	33	20	53	13	11	24
	Play–Indoor	22	17	39	10	13	23
	Outdoor	16	3	19	3	7	10
	Unusual Situations	0	4	4	0	0	0
	Totals	124	86	210	46	39	85
Emilie	Sleep	8	5	13	2	3	5
	Dressing	9	11	20	8	3	11
	Washing	10	6	16	1	4	5
	Toilet	17	8	25	3	6	9
	Eating	32	21	53	13	11	24
	Play–Indoor	15	19	34	7	7	14
	Outdoor	34	9	43	1	4	5
	Unusual Situations	1	3	4	0	1	1
	Totals	126	82	208	35	39	74

Continues . . .

Figure 7.2 Continued

Child	Routines	1st Half	2nd Half	Total Period	'1st Half	2nd Half	Total Period
Marie	Sleep	16	9	25	5	10	15
	Dressing	12	14	26	10	7	17
	Washing	11	3	14	2	2	4
	Toilet	18	15	33	4	5	9
	Eating	33	17	50	13	14	27
	Play–Indoor	31	10	41	15	7	22
	Outdoor	45	4	49	4	11	15
	Unusual Situations	2	1	3	0	3	3
	Totals	168	73	241	53	59	112
Yvonne	Sleep	13	11	24	6	3	9
	Dressing	6	10	16	7	3	10
	Washing	10	7	17	3	3	6
	Toilet	35	13	48	1	3	4
	Eating	29	27	56	10	11	21
	Play–Indoor	30	22	52	13	8	21
	Outdoor	36	3	39	10	7	17
	Unusual Situations	1	2	3	0	0	0
	Totals	160	95	255	50	38	88

Source: MacArthur and Ford (1937)

Dionne warned Dafoe that Premier Hepburn was being apprised of Blatz's unauthorised actions in managing the nursery, and that Dionne was mobilising the Ontario French Canadian Education Association in this cause.[41] Oliva's French Canadian nationalism was, however, to some degree merely instrumental: at a guardians' meeting in January of 1940, Dionne seconded a motion to ask the Department of Education to teach English to the quintuplets, 'in view of the business manager's statement that a loss of revenue was caused by the Quintuplets' inability to speak English'.[42]

Revenue was also not far from the thoughts of the scientists themselves: Dr Blatz and his collaborators were paid $600 to reimburse them for expenses relating to the scientific conference on the quintuplets, and Blatz's Toronto nursery billed the fund for at least $1,380 for 'expenses re research and consultation'.[43] The interesting practice of billing one's subjects for research expenses is perhaps an indication that the scientists regarded the quintuplets as a crown corporation with an unlimited expense account. Following in the footsteps of both the biological father and the political collective father, science was engaged in a paradoxical move to gain ownership of the quintuplet set but have the institution finance its own takeover.

While science, in the person of Dr Blatz and his team, exercised control over the quintuplets for a couple of years, another powerful institution exercised life-long control and some forms of ownership, namely the media. The newspapers, photo syndicates, and radio stations were probably the most powerful agency in the lives of the girls, exercising power over all other would-be owners. The relations of the government with the parents, for instance, were largely mediated by the newspapers, since in the early days of the guardianship the Premier and other officials met with Dafoe regularly but not with the parents. Oliva Dionne, whose English (unlike Elzire's) was excellent, learned to call the local press and make his demands on the government through the pages of the newspaper. Furthermore, while the girls did not always know what scientists or cabinet ministers said about them, they did know how the media portrayed them, and, in the absence of normal contact with peers and adults, their direct and indirect contacts with photographers and reporters were virtually the only mirror on which they could see themselves as social actors. While 2 or 3 years old, the girls saw Fred Davis, the photographer who had exclusive rights to their pictures, much more regularly than they saw their parents. While the right of the government to control the girls was often contested, the 'natural' right of the media (usually spoken about as 'the right of the public') to direct the girls' lives went unchallenged. The quintuplets' own account criticises everyone from parents to doctors to government officials, but not the media (Brough, 1965). The representation of the girls provided by a New York songwriter's lyrics would not have surprised the girls (or the guardians, or the parents):

Who are the girls whose pictures appear in the papers
   for us to see –
Annette, Emilie, Cecile, Yvonne and Marie
And who are the girls who are knocking them dead
   with popularity?
Annette, Emilie, Cecile, Yvonne and Marie. . . .

They'll win the fight we know and their names and fame
  will live in history
Now their bottles and their battles and their games and
  nursery rhymes
Are depicted in The Telegram, The Journal, News and Times.

(Musician Pat Gleason to Wilson, 22 April 1937,
'General' file, Box 3, DQG)

Although some of the ways in which the media lay claim to public
figures are not easily contested, the guardians went out of their
way to increase the media's power by selling the right to represent
the quintuplets to large American syndicates. As long as the girls
never left the nursery, and were thus easily posed for the cameras
at the reporters' convenience and without hindrance from parents
or siblings, the problems were not apparent (to the guardians; they
may have been apparent to some nurses). But an unprecedented
trip to Toronto for the quintuplets to meet their legal/symbolic
father, the King, brought matters to a head. As the logistics of the
trip were being worked out by top-level officials, the Attorney
General, realising that no amount of security could prevent
unauthorised photographs from being taken during this trip,
asked for a legal opinion on possible lawsuits by the corporations
holding exclusive rights of representation. He decided that despite
the strong possibility of lawsuits, the trip ought to go ahead. But
as he had foreseen, the vast police detail failed to prevent all
manner of photographers from snapping pictures of the hitherto
recluse quintuplets.[44]
  Predictably, the photo syndicate, NEA, initiated a suit for breach
of contract, telling the guardians that:

any removal of the Quintuplets from the hospital in which they
were kept would, insofar as the contract between the Guardians
and NEA Service Inc. was concerned, be entirely at the Guardians'
risk and that if any photographs or sketches of the Quintuplets
should be made by anyone other than NEA Service Inc., NEA
Service Inc. could only regard that as a breach of its contract.

(President of NEA to Guardians, 24 May 1939,
'NEA' file, Box 9, DQG)

That NEA should regard healthy 5-year-old girls as dumb animals
who ought not to be 'removed' from 'the hospital in which they

were kept' is perhaps not surprising, but it is noteworthy that the legal power of the press syndicates to keep the girls literally imprisoned was not directly challenged.

Absorbed in the details of these epic battles, one might neglect to ask who was excluded from the arena before the battle began. When one notices the gender composition of the titans, however, the absence of maternal contestants is striking. The government, the media, science and medicine shared a predominant ethnic and class basis, one challenged by the minority Francophone community and by the father. With regard to both gender composition and gender ideology, however, these warring factions were, one might say, united to a man. Contemporaries were so transfixed by the unusual phenomenon of competition among fathers that they completely overlooked the absence, or more accurately the suppression, of maternal discourse. In the mid-1930s neither French nor English Canada had a strong women's movement; such a movement would have given Mrs Dionne both a political base for a public claim distinct from her husband's and a language in which to formulate it.

As mentioned earlier, Mrs Dionne did try to mobilise the female wing of the ruling Liberal Party in support of her claim. In a speech that annoyed the government, a leader of the Ontario Women's Liberal Association reported that she had talked with Mrs Dionne 'in my own language as a French woman, as one Northerner to another, and as one mother to another'. She then challenged the government to unite what she called 'the family' (in contrast to the 'two families' discussed in the guardians' correspondence).[45] But even this ally did not go so far as to directly support Mrs Dionne's demand to add her and two other mothers to the board of guardians. Having failed to enter the real seat of power, Mrs Dionne seems to have turned her considerable energies to fighting not the fatherly government but her direct rivals, the nurses. Throughout 1938 and 1939, the nurse's log and Mrs Dionne's letters document the pitched battles for the affection of the girls fought among women in the nursery as men struggled for ownership in the more overtly public world outside. The sordid details of these battles need not be described here; the general strategy is clear from a letter of Mrs Dionne to the Official Guardian:

> Nurse [A] incites my children against me as well as against their father. She teaches them to despise and have contempt for me . . . she has a nefarious influence in the lives of the little ones.

Imagine the deadly feelings planted by the girl as she told the quintuplets not to love their father and mother because they are too dirty. I don't sleep at night, when I think that this stranger is corrupting my children's hearts.

(Mrs Dionne to Wilson, 26 July 1939,
'Mrs Dionne' file, Box 2, DQG;
translation from French by author)

The association of the biological parents with dirt went back some years. When the girls had been small babies, Mrs Dionne and the rest of the commoner family had been forced by Dr Dafoe to wear masks and gowns when visiting the quintuplets, whereas the official photographer and visiting dignitaries such as Premier Hepburn were presumed to be germ-free.[46] Even if Dr Dafoe was originally responsible for this selective germ theory, its enforcement was the responsibility of the female staff.[47] A letter from Oliva Dionne's lawyer to Wilson describes an allegedly typical skirmish in the battles among maternal figures:

Mrs Dionne said to Emilie: 'Why don't you come to see your mama? What is the matter? Don't you love your mama?' And Emilie answered, 'No, I don't love mama, neither Papa, because they are dirty. [Nurse B] said so. No, never, never love mama nor papa, love only [the nurses] and doctor.'

(H. Saint-Jacques to Wilson, 24 July 1939,
'Saint-Jacques' file, Box 8, DQG)

Legally excluded, and physically and emotionally marginalised from her children's lives, Mrs Dionne was certainly one of the prime victims of the guardianship. And yet, the attempts by well-meaning chroniclers to portray her as a natural mother with unambiguous natural love for the quintuplets are not free from ideological assumptions. Pop historian Pierre Berton, defending the honour of the devoutly Catholic rural family against the perfidious state, writes that 'childbearing was to her a process as natural as eating' (Berton, 1977: 24). But this claim is undermined by his own account of the words uttered by Elzire Dionne as she realised she was giving birth to five babies: 'What will the neighbours say? They will think we are pigs' (Berton, 1977: 76). Mrs Dionne may well have regarded her peculiar fertility as a sign of sexual corruption, and the quintuplets' birth as a modern-day monstrous birth. Childbearing is, like eating, always culturally constructed, and it is possible that the cultural frameworks available to Mrs Dionne led her to regard the babies, who were in any case neither nursed nor changed by her, with greater-than-average maternal ambivalence. In their infancy, the girls had lacked a constant caretaker, a mother or mother-substitute against whom they might define their individuality. They were burdened by a surfeit of fathers, of course, but these fathers acted as absentee owners. With the press as their only mirror, it is perhaps not surprising that rather than speak in the first person (either the common 'I' or the royal 'we') they learned to refer to themselves in the third person collective, not as 'we' but as 'les jumelles', or, more curiously, 'les Quints'.[48] Their self-designation as 'les Quints' clearly reveals that although speaking in French, they took up the English word, coined by the media and copyrighted by the government, which marked them as non-children, as the unique world attraction.

But what were the possible alternative discourses available at the time to understand the phenomenon of 'the quintuplets'? One might speculate what might have happened if the Dionne quintuplets, rather than be immediately constituted as tourist attractions and media stars, had been regarded as cases for Children's Aid or other social workers. Such apparently child-centred discourses may have dealt with the girls through the admittedly modern and problematic social identity of 'the child' – although, given the scientific uniqueness of identical quintuplets, it is difficult to imagine that the girls could ever have been treated as 'children' and not as a separate and exotic species. Although the girls' self-perception was, of course, peculiarly warped by the lens of the Quintuplet–Quintland institution, well-meaning psychologists or social workers attempting to make the girls 'ordinary' would not in all likelihood have provided the conditions for the girls to see themselves as subjects instead of objects. Medicine, sociology, psychology and pedagogy might have eliminated the crassest forms of exploitation, but, as seen in Dr Blatz's childrearing plan, modern forms of discipline are often more intrusive than the old-fashioned exhibition of 'freak' children at carnivals.

Apart from psychological discourses on child welfare, which as we have seen entered the girls' lives far less than one might expect, an alternative strategy might have been to mobilise the rhetoric of natural motherhood to justify leaving the children on the farm.

This type of rhetoric, however appealing, would have been difficult to implement given the fact that by the mid-1930s Canadian women could not escape the practices and discourses organising maternity on modern lines (Arnup, 1990; Strong-Boag, 1988). More importantly, a mother who already had five children could not very well assume sole care for five tiny newborns, and community resources, although very useful for a few weeks of crisis, could hardly cope with the long-term challenge, especially given the Depression. The very real physical fragility of the newborn girls made it in any case difficult to rely on common sense and tradition. The 'traditional' women in and around the Dionne household could not in good conscience reject the frozen breast milk and the incubators shipped by rail from metropolitan centres. Would an insistence on natural motherhood have perhaps resulted in a tragedy of a different order for the girls? And how would a female-centred discourse of motherhood have differed from traditional Catholic gender ideology?

Regardless of which definition of motherhood is chosen out of the range available at the time, maternal discourses of whatever type might also have 'failed' the girls. Feminist writers on family law sometimes forget that children have interests which do not always coincide with those of their mother. Even if a maternal presence, either individual or collective, either traditional or modern, had been able to make itself felt, the children might still have become pawns in a battle for ownership, one now including maternal contestants. Nevertheless, even if inclusion of maternal discourses would not necessarily have given the girls a chance to represent themselves rather than be constantly represented by others, it would at least have acknowledged the gender of those who actually did the work of childrearing. It seemed in fact that the less work one performed, the better chance one had of gaining legal power over the children. This was certainly the case for the powerful paternal provincial government, which neither did any child-rearing nor (despite its claims) paid for it to be done. The provincial government managed simultaneously to appear beneficent and to generate revenues from the alleged object of beneficence. From the standpoint of administration, the guardianship of the quintuplets was a brilliant example of financially creative social regulation.

Analysing the government's practices regarding the quin-tuplets, their guardians, their parents, and their money, suggests that social regulation is best understood not as the control of already distinct areas of social activity but rather as a process which first constitutes the object to be administered. The government's actions constituted a group of human beings not as 'children', as one might have expected, but as a nationally owned resource. Family, gender, ethnicity, and childrearing were all regulated in important ways by the Ontario government's actions regarding the quintuplets, but these were indirect effects of resource management. This shows that there is no pre-given distinct sphere of childrearing which is then managed in various ways by various agencies: rather, regulatory activity sets out the criteria for what is and is not a children's issue, and even what is or is not a child.[49] The legal and administrative practices governing the girls' lives do not therefore shed much light on the fate of other children. The sisters lived as icons of childhood, representing that which they could not experience.

ACKNOWLEDGEMENTS

Many thanks are due to Ian McKay, Carol Smart and Cynthia Wright for their careful reading of an earlier draft. Cynthia also contributed many insights and bits of quint-knowledge. Ki Namaste collected the newspaper articles.

This chapter is dedicated to the memory of my son Daniel Valverde (1989–90), whose first stirrings were its inspiration.

NOTES

1 Official Guardian of Ontario, Dionne Quintuplet Guardianship materials (Box 1–12 of Series 4–53, RG 4, Public Archives of Ontario; referred to as DQG for short).
2 Dr Dafoe explained that the Francophone farmers among whom he practised were a people 'of Norman descent, rugged and virile . . . Race suicide [i.e. birth control] is non-existent' (Dr A.R. Dafoe (1934) 'The Dionne Quintuplets', *Journal of the American Medical Association* 103: 673, 1 Sept.
3 Ottawa officials wanted to tax the trust fund as a single entity, but the Official Guardian, probably thinking that splitting it in five would mean a lower tax rate, fought this successfully. See 'Income Tax' file, Box 4, DQG; and Minutes of March 1940 meeting of the Guardians, 'Minutes' file, Box 6, DQG. It is noteworthy that the 'Income Tax' file is much thicker than any other file in the records, including education-or health-related files.

4 See Box 182 of the Hepburn papers (RG 3, Public Archives of Ontario). The Dafoe Papers also contain relevant letters, though many of these seek medical advice and thus use the quintuplets as a pretext to obtain free services.

5 See the scrapbook of press clippings in the A.R. Dafoe papers, Public Archives of Ontario.

6 'Agreement between Oliva Dionne and Chicago World's Fair promoters' 31 May 1934: p. 1 vol. 1, Series C, Dafoe Papers, Public Archives of Ontario. By 1935 the infamous contract had long lapsed, but a trip to Chicago by Mr and Mrs Dionne re-activated the issue, since the Chicago promoters threatened to sue the parents and the province for their breach of the 1934 agreement.

7 'Roebuck breaks Chicago contract' *Globe* 27 July 1934; see also the almost identical article in the *Toronto Star*, same date. Both the *Globe* and the *Telegram* published editorials on 28 July supporting the Attorney General's action.

8 Undated report, probably late 1938, in 'Reports of Official Guardian' file, Box 8, DQG.

9 'Province plans full care for whole Dionne family', *Star* 27 March 1935: 23.

10 'An Act Respecting the Guardianship of the Dionne Quintuplets', 1st session, 19th Legislature, Ontario, 25 George V, 1935.

11 'Dionne family to get care' *Mail and Empire* 27 March 1935: 11.

12 See newspaper coverage of the legislature debates, in the *Star* and the *Mail and Empire* 14–27 March 1935.

13 'Animosity flares over quints' future' *Globe* 15 March 1935: 11.

14 Next to an article soothingly entitled 'Province Plans Full Care for Whole Dionne Family' (*Star* 27 March 1935: 23), an article titled 'Highest Birth Among the Unemployed' stated that in the US relief authorities were contemplating severe measures to deal with the excess fertility of parents on relief.

15 'Dionne Bill Being Aimed at Chisellers' *Globe* 12 March 1935.

16 The Ontario Provincial Police did investigate a 1937 rumour of a kidnapping plot which was quickly revealed to be a hoax. (File 1.4, Series E-103, RG 23). Given the thoroughness of the police investigation of 1937 and its full documentation in the archival files, one cannot help but wonder if the 1935 threat was concocted by government officials to boost their claim.

17 'FEAR PLAN TO SPIRIT QUINTUPLETS TO U. S.' *Star* 25 March 1935: 1. In the early 1940s, a proposed trip to the US was also described through the discourse of kingly fatherhood: 'The Guardians now propose to transport the five little ambassadors on a special train to Washington, escorted by the Hon. Mitchell Hepburn, Prime Minister of the Province of Ontario, who will introduce the wards of his Majesty King George VI to President Roosevelt.' Undated document titled 'Proposed draft statement to be issued by the Official Guardian', 'Visit to US' file, Box 8, DQG.

18 Although contacted initially, the Children's Aid had declined to be

involved because in its judgement (probably stated by local northern officials) there was no child neglect.

19 In the 1910s freak shows at the Canadian National Exhibition in Toronto regularly included children; see e.g. the photograph and caption of Siamese twins, 'A Wonderful Exhibit' *Toronto Daily News* 5 September 1911: 5.

20 'Dionne Bill Being Aimed at Chisellers', *Globe* 12 March 1935.

21 'Mother of Quints Voices Complaint' *Globe* 28 March 1935: 12.

22 See memo from Wilson to Hepburn and to the Attorney General, 3 May 1937, 'Reports of the Official Guardian' file, Box 8, DQG.

23 A touching instance of father-to-father bonding is found in a letter from Wilson to Munro written as the government was preparing to give the quintuplets to their (biological) father:

> Sometime I really would like to write you and tell you just how much I appreciate your continuing assistance to me in the Guardianship. I will only say now that to me it is the one feature that has come through with colours – that is our mutual co-operation and friendship and the basic loyalty to the cause which we will endeavour to serve.

One wonders whether either man would have been able to precisely name the cause to which they were so dedicated. (Wilson to Munro, 1 April 1944, 'Munro' file, Box 6, DQG.)

24 On Wilson's extra pay, see letter from Wilson to Attorney General Leslie Blackwell, 3 October 1944, in 'Surrogate Court Audits' file, Box 9, DQG. The extent of the expenses charged by Wilson to the trust fund can be gauged from the large collection of bills deposited in Box 11, DQG. Guardian Judge Valin also collected $600 in excess of his pension as compensation for time spent passing accounts. In total, there were about 20 people on the monthly payroll of the Guardianship.

25 Valin was seen by the nationalist Francophones as overly assimilated; see Frederick Edwards, 'The Quints Question' *Maclean's* 15 July 1941: 41.

26 Wilson's memo [probably to Attorney General], 20 June 1941, 'Reports of the Official Guardian' file, Box 8, DQG.

27 Wilson's memo [probably to the Attorney General], June 20 1941, 'Reports of the Official Guardian' file, Box 8, DQG

28 Francis Talbot (1941) 'The Quints are Seven – and Want to Go Home' *America* 16 August; Lillian Barker (1941) 'Dionne Wins Back the Quints', *America* 25 October: 65.

29 Memo by Wilson dated 20 June 1941, 'Reports of the Official Guardian' file, Box 8, DQG.

30 Ontario's Francophone daily painted a romanticised picture of a suddenly enlarged patriarchal family in which nobody was allowed to talk at dinner by order of the father and in which everyone got up at 6.30 a.m. and enjoyed the outdoors; see 'Les Dionnelles retrouvent la vraie vie de famille' *Le Droit* 27 May 1944.

31 Auditor's report, 31 March 1937, in 'Reports of the Official Guardian' file, Box 8, DQG; 'Quints Pay Cash for War Bonds', *North Bay Nugget* 15 January 1940: 1.

32 F. Edwards, 'The Quint Question' *Macleans* 15 July 1941: 37.
33 Minutes of special meeting held in North Bay, 20 July 1938, in 'Minutes' file, Box 6, DQG. (For a detailed description and pictures of Quintland, see Berton, 1977: Chapter 10.)
34 Minutes of January 1940 meeting of guardians, 'Minutes' file, Box 6, DQG; see letter from guardianship secretary to the provincial Department of Education, included in the minutes of the guardians' meeting in April 1941.
35 Frederick Edwards, 'The Quint Question', *Macleans* 15 July 1941; Berton (1977: 244 ff.).
36 Wilson, Memo dated 4 April 1941, 'Minutes' file, Box 6, DQG.
37 'Hair' file, Box 3, DQG; see also Minutes of guardians' meeting for November 1940, and memo dated 4 April 1941, both in 'Minutes' file, Box 6, DQG.
38 Edwards, 'The Quint Question': 36 (see note 32).
39 Frank Donovan to Munro, 14 May 1941, 'Pathé' file, Box 8, DQG.
40 'Looking into the Future with Mrs Dionne', speech given by Mrs J. Poupure on 27 November 1937 to the Ontario Women's Liberal Association; copy of the speech in 'Mrs Dionne' file, Box 2, DQG.
41 Oliva Dionne to Dr Dafoe, 26 February 1938, Series C, Volume 3, Dafoe Papers, Public Archives of Ontario. The Association passed a resolution calling for French Catholic educators for the Dionne girls (to which the official guardian agreed, fearing ethnic battles) and for the reunification of the Dionne family (to which Wilson did not yet agree). See letter from the Association (ACFEO) to Wilson, 19 March 1939, 'Education' file, Box 3, DQG.
42 Guardians to Ontario Department of Education, 18 January 1940, 'Education' file, Box 3 DQG; see also Oliva Dionne to Wilson, 5 March 1941, asking for an English teacher (same file).
43 Minutes of guardians' meetings, January 1938 and October 1937, 'Minutes' file, Box 5, DQG.
44 Attorney General G.D. Conant to the guardianship's main lawyer, R.L. Kellock, 11 April 1939, in 'Pathé' file, Box 8, DQG.
45 'Looking into the future with Mrs Dionne', 'Mrs Dionne' file, Box 2, DQG.
46 'Mother of Quints voices complaint', *Globe* 28 March 1935: 12; see also Berton (1977:119).
47 See the nurse's log for June–September 1939, untitled file, Box 11, DQG.
48 The phrase 'les Quints', reportedly from the girls' mouths, is found in Frederick Edwards, 'The Quints Question', *Macleans* 15 July 1941: 8–9 and 34–8; 'les jumelles' in Talbot, 'The Quints are Seven': 511 and Barker 'Dionne Wins Back the Girls': 65. (See note 28.)
49 A few years after the Dionne quintuplets' birth, the Supreme Court of Canada was called upon to adjudicate the question of what constituted a child, for the purposes of an amount of money left in his will by an eccentric Toronto lawyer to the woman who had the most children in 10 years. The court eventually decided that neither stillbirths nor healthy, illegitimate children counted as children (Orkin, 1981).

Chapter 7

Whose property?
The double standard of adultery in nineteenth-century law

Ursula Vogel

'In the ancient world adultery refers originally to the man who breaks into another man's marriage, and to the woman who breaks the bonds of her own; adultery violates the proprietary rights of a husband over his wife' (Delling, 1959: 666).

INTRODUCTION

In March 1990 the German press reported on a case of adultery tried before a disciplinary court of the American army. It involved a black woman soldier who was accused of sexual relations with a married man, an officer with the same contingent. German observers expressed their incredulity at the fact that actions of this kind could still be brought before the law long after adultery had ceased to be a criminal offence. The woman was eventually expelled from the army; her partner was posted with another regiment but suffered no further adverse consequences (*Berliner Tageszeitung*, 24 March 1990). At about the same time newspapers carried the story of a Saudi princess who was found guilty of adultery and stoned to death (her partner was executed). It was not only the severity of the punishment that attracted attention but the fact that under Islamic law a husband could not be accused of the same crime. In England observers, in the 1950s, might have witnessed the occasional application of legal procedures – dating back to Anglo-Saxon times – through which a wronged husband could claim damages from the lover of his wife. Again, remedies of this sort would not have been available to a wife in the reverse case of her husband's adultery (Smart, 1984: 42).

These examples contain the vestiges of a long and powerful legal tradition which has created 'adultery' as an offence of different quality and consequence for women and men. Stated in most general terms, adultery refers to a sexual relationship between a married person and someone other than the legitimate spouse. Neutral definitions of this kind are, however, bound to obscure the fundamental asymmetry at the very core of the normative construction of adultery. In the pre-Christian world, notably in Roman law, which so profoundly influenced European legal history, only a wife was capable of committing adultery (i.e. of breaking the marriage bond). The very same act on the part of her husband had no name in the language of the law, as long as he did not violate the marriage of another man (Delling, 1959; Lerner, 1986).

This partiality of the law is commonly referred to as the 'double standard'. If we search for the reasons that can explain the double optic of moral and legal norms, we will encounter, in one form or other, a recurring theme – cited here in the words of a seventeenth-century English aristocrat whose successful petition to the House of Lords for a divorce from his adulterous wife invoked the 'common privilege of every freeman in the world to have an heir of his own body to inherit what he possessed either of honour or estate' (McGregor, 1957: 10).

The idea that a wife's (but not a husband's) adultery strikes at the order of property and, as a direct consequence, at the foundations of civil society itself, reflects a near-unanimous consensus of legislators, jurists, moralists echoed over many centuries of European legal history. Whose property is at issue here? And what kind of proprietary interests have to be guarded against female adultery? Why does a woman's infidelity, but not a man's, have a distinctly political dimension and relevance? These are the questions that my chapter will address.

Both historically and conceptually, we often refer to the constitution of patriarchy in terms of proprietary power and interests. The focus on adultery allows us to identify the several and ambivalent meanings that are bound up in this language of property. The rights that the adulterous woman violates refer to different claims as well as different claimants. They refer to a man's ownership of children, to his control over property (estates) and lineage, and to his right of exclusive access to the wife's body and sexuality. But it is not only the property right of a private person that is at stake here, but the collective interest of society represented by the state. In most legal systems of the past we will find adultery at a strategic intersection of private and public law. As a violation of the rights of particular individuals, it calls upon the civil law to adjudicate property claims, custody of children and other consequences of divorce or separation. At the same time adultery counts as a punishable offence under the criminal law, which will exact retribution for the violation of the public interest. We shall see that it is the normative order of this second domain which, in modern justifications of the double standard, establishes the particular gravity and incommensurate quality of a wife's infidelity. In modern civil law ownership rights in another person, epitomised in the relations of slavery and of feudal servitude, fall outside the category of legitimate property. But although indefensible on grounds of individual entitlement, the husband's right to the wife's body retains the appearance of legitimacy because it is sheltered by claims made on behalf of the public good.

This chapter will trace the political construction of the double standard of adultery in the marriage law of the *Code Napoléon* (1804) and in the public debates about divorce that took place in nineteenth-century Germany and England. In much of the literature the double standard is cited as if it required no further explication, as if it were but the continuous re-enactment of some permanent disposition of human nature. But as Thomas's important essay (1959) has shown, the meaning of what may appear a timeless code of sexual morality is intimately bound up with the historically specific and changing pattern of a society's legal and political institutions, with its religious traditions, and with the interests and values of particular groups. We will find that in our period the much-invoked authority of an undisrupted legal tradition is deceptive. The invention of such a tradition was itself part of political strategies propelled by the force of the European reaction against the principles of the French Revolution. In France, the reaction sought to paralyse the emancipatory potential released by the civil legislation of the revolutionary assemblies between 1789 and 1795; in Prussia it turned against the legacies of Enlightenment rationalism that had inspired the liberal divorce law of the civil code of 1794. In England, legal developments followed an altogether different route. But here, too, the special status of women's adultery – affirmed in the Matrimonial Causes Act of 1857 – can be related to a dialectical process of modernisation and reaction. Here, as in Germany and France, the entrenchment of the double standard in modern law was a response to the liberalisation of divorce and, in particular, to the feared consequences of women's sexual freedom. Considered by its wider historical implications it was a reaction against the uncontrollable dynamic and the uncertain costs of political modernisation. To reinforce the security of sexual property at the centre of the marriage relation was a way of controlling this process – and a way of shifting its costs.

THE CODE NAPOLÉON

Not only in its own time but for more than a century after it was first enacted (1804) the French *Code civil* was celebrated as the unsurpassed model of a modern legal system. It expressed the unity and power of the nation state; it was the spearhead of economic and social progress and the guarantor of the revolutionary idea of equal citizenship. However, if we turn to the law of marriage we find that it was not part of this universe of modern legal principles. On the contrary, cast into the nexus of obedience and protection (*Code civil*, 213) the relationship between wife and husband retained the very structures of an ascribed hierarchical order that the bourgeois revolution had excised from all other spheres of the private law (Portemer, 1962; Holthöfer, 1982; Schnapper, 1987; Gerhard, 1988). The code affirmed the unquestionable authority of the husband and father as ruler of the 'royauté domestique' (Holthöfer, 1982: 435). Conjugal rights and obligations followed from the central presumption of the married woman's *incapacité*. She was, to summarise briefly, incapable of any legally valid action unless explicitly authorised by her husband (or, in exceptional cases, by a judge). She could neither conclude contracts nor engage in business or paid work outside the home, nor make any dispositions with regard to her property. The *puissance maritale* entitled the husband to control her correspondence, to watch over her friends, to call upon the coercive power of the state (the police) to return her to his home. The nature and origin of this power are nowhere more clearly revealed than in the rules prescribed for divorce proceedings:

> The husband can demand a divorce on the ground of his wife's adultery. The wife can demand a divorce on the ground of the

husband's adultery if he has lived with his concubine under the roof of the matrimonial home.

(*Code civil*: 229, 230)

Historically, these rules derived directly from the customary laws of the Ancien Régime (Portemer, 1962). But the very act of restating them was both expression and vehicle of 'reactionary' politics. The marriage law of the Napoleonic Code embodied the claim of the post-revolutionary state to be the sole legislator and arbiter in a domain that had for centuries been under the doctrinal and jurisdictional supremacy of the Catholic church. In preserving the obligatory civil marriage and, albeit with significant restrictions, the legitimacy of divorce the code built upon the foundations laid by the *droit intermédiaire*, the civil legislation of the revolutionary period. At the same time, and with no less determination, it aimed to rein back the dangerous egalitarian consequences of a revolution that had gone too far.

Stated briefly, between 1789 and 1795 it had been the intention of the legislators to rebuild the whole system of private law on the principles of individual liberty and equality (Sagnac, 1898). To achieve the goal of a uniform, secular citizenship it was necessary to release individuals from the traditional impositions of both natural and conventional distinctions; to incorporate Protestants, Jews and aliens into the legal community; to free the peasants and their land from the fetters of feudal servitude; and, similarly, to liberate the members of the family from the despotism of the husband and father. The law of 20 September 1792 created both the *état civil* and the obligatory civil marriage: '*Le moyen âge disparaissait. La philosophie triomphait*' (Sagnac, 1898: 275). The most radical step in the sequence of reforms followed from the new understanding of marriage as but an ordinary civil contract, namely the legalisation of divorce (Conrad, 1950).

If the legitimacy of divorce was claimed as the indispensable condition of general liberty, it was also seen to confer particular benefits on women. As long as the prevailing marriage laws still committed women to a status of legal incapacity and submission, divorce offered them the only route of exit by which they could escape from marital despotism. The most remarkable and truly revolutionary features of the law of 1792 lay both in the unprecedented extension of the causes that enabled the marriage partners to seek divorce and in the fact that these were to be available on equal conditions to wife and husband (Traer, 1980). A marriage could be dissolved upon mutual consent and even on one partner's allegation of *incompatibilité d'humeur*. Adultery as such no longer figured among the abuses of conjugal obligations. It was incorporated into a more general clause of *'dérèglement de moeurs notoire'* (Sagnac, 1898: 246). Since the charge of a 'notorious offence against morality' could be claimed by either spouse against the other, and since the custody of children was to be decided on strictly equal grounds, the demise of the double standard seemed assured.

Under the significant shift of political intentions that followed on the reign of terror and the anarchic state of the French republic after 1795 the permissiveness of the divorce law – and the soaring number of divorce cases many of which were initiated by women (Phillips, 1980) – appeared as the very symbol of a society in disarray. And it became the dominant concern of the jurists entrusted with the further development of the civil code to revoke the excessive liberty granted to individuals under the law of 1792. In order to break the link between contractual freedom and divorce legislators stressed the special nature of the marriage contract, its higher purposes and the enduring commitments that set it apart from ordinary civil contracts (*Conférence* 1805(12)). As a matter of general moral principle, the contraction of individual freedom that this argument sought to vindicate was to bear equally on men and women. But when formulated in terms of institutional safeguards, the burden came to fall on women. The very problem of anchoring marriage in indisputable principles of order and permanence without returning it to the domain of religion was solved at their expense. On the one hand, the law had to assume the purely secular status of marriage (as the necessary condition of the state's exclusive jurisdiction). On the other hand, there was a need to establish some equivalent of the disciplinary power once guaranteed by the sacramental status of marriage. The code reconciled the conflicting demands of order and freedom by reinstating the husband's proprietary rights to the wife's person and by attaching severe penalties to the violation of these rights.

The most striking change in the *Code Napoléon* brought back the full rigour of the double standard of adultery: that *'distinction honorable et utile'* (Sagnac, 1898: 375). Although the letter of the law seemed to bind both spouses to an obligation of mutual fidelity, it licensed in the husband's case a 'state of virtual polygamy' (Schleifer, 1972: 98). The same law that entitled him to sue for divorce on the evidence of the wife's adultery took no notice of his extra-marital affairs unless he had gone as far as to entertain an adulterous relationship in the matrimonial home. Unequal treatment of a similar magnitude also prevailed when the case was carried into the domain of the criminal law. A wife convicted of adultery was to be sent to prison or a house of correction for a period ranging from 3 months to 2 years. In the reverse case, and only under the aggravating circumstances cited above, the husband had to pay a fine of between 100 and 2,000 francs. A similar penalty was imposed on the partner of the adulterous woman. Moreover, if a husband had in revenge killed or gravely injured the wife, the law would concede the mitigating circumstances of a *délit d'honneur*. Needless to say that no such concessions were available to the wife.

What reasons can account for the 'unprecedented rigour and cruelty' (Sagnac, 1898: 374) with which the French code turned against the wife? Why did the full force of the reaction express itself in the recriminalisation of female adultery? From the deliberations that took place at the drafting stage two main lines of argument emerge that consider the moral implications of sexual difference, on the one hand, and the demands of the republic, on the other. They converge in the link between certain paternity and *'la tranquillité publique'* (*Conférence* 1805(12): 122). That the wife's adultery might result in a 'foreign child' usurping the husband's property (*Conférence* 1805(2): 180) and that as a consequence the order of society itself would descend into anarchy, this projection was made to resemble a self-evident truth. But, as such, it was strangely out of tune with the foundational principles of the code itself. That is, private property that the code established as the norm of ownership did no longer have the meaning to which the paternity–public-order link had once owed its functional symmetry. In the agrarian society of feudalism where each cell was rooted in the heritage of landed property marriage was the site of strategic alliances between families who in turn acted as but the representatives or stewards of their property. In this historical environment marriage served exclusively the function of guaranteeing legitimate offspring and the perpetuity of the lineage. The chastity of women was traded as a good in a complex system of exchanges designed to transmit estates, glory and honour to future generations (Duby, 1988).

The order of private property guaranteed by the *Code Napoléon* was of a different kind. It presumed the unconstrained right of each individual to dispose over his property and the mobility, transferability and partibility of all goods. Indeed, in those parts of the marriage law that dealt with the regulation of matrimonial property, the legislator left the parties free to make their own arrangements. They might, for example, opt for a separation of goods which gave to women some degree of freedom in administering and controlling their property. This freedom was, however, bounded by a non-negotiable condition: no property regime could be chosen that would impinge on the rights resulting from the *'puissance maritale sur la personne de la femme'* (*Code civil*: 1388). The barrier was justified by the different imperatives of the private and the public sphere. Individual liberty might reign in the domain of economic goods and interests. The public order rested on the principle of undisputed authority in state and family alike (*Conférence* 1805(5)). The basis of the husband's rule was only secure to the extent that it could be fortified against the wife's freedom over her own body. Ownership rights of a kind that could not be found in any other sphere of the civil law survived in marriage. The atavistic character of these rights and the vacuum of legitimacy in which they operated were concealed by their alleged relevance to the public interest.

But, what was the public interest as distinct from men's interest? What special claim did the public or the state have on women's fidelity? The texts give no answer to these questions. The proprietary claims of husband and state are locked together in a circular process of legitimation in which each refers to the other and neither stands justified.

THE DUAL STANDARD OF ADULTERY – THE HONOUR OF THE FEMALE SEX: THE DEBATE ON THE DIVORCE LAWS IN NINETEENTH-CENTURY PRUSSIA

In subordinating women to special laws of a more exacting sexual morality the framers of the French Code claimed the imperatives of state interest. In Prussia, the partisans of the political reaction which gathered momentum after the Napoleonic wars (Buchholz,

1979) pursued similar objectives. Here, too, the aim was to rebuild the moral foundations of state authority from the centre of an authoritarian marriage rendered secure by the wife's special obligation of chastity. But the language in which these aims were stated differed remarkably. While the formulations of the Napoleonic code left no doubt that women's fidelity was to be secured in a relationship of power and subjection, German jurists converted the nexus of enforced inequality into an affirmation of female dignity.

The crusade to restore the indissolubility of marriage and to reinforce the criminal dimensions of adultery as an offence against the public order was, in the case of German jurisprudence, aimed at the divorce laws of the Prussian civil code (1794). A product of enlightened absolutism, this code combined the paternalist intentions of the autocratic state and the philosophical legacies of eighteenth-century rationalism. In placing person and property of the wife under the husband's guardianship the marriage law followed the traditional hierarchical model of ascribed status and differential obligations (Gerhard, 1978; Vogel, 1988). But the formulation of concrete duties – which owed much to the contractual premises and egalitarian implications of eighteenth-century natural law – tended to emphasise the joint responsibilities of husband and wife and the mutual character of conjugal commitments. This applied in particular to the obligation of fidelity and to the roughly equal consequences that followed upon its violation. The contractual foundations of conjugal right were most evident in the provisions for terminating the marriage bond. The code permitted divorce not only on the traditional grounds of adultery, malicious desertion and excessive violence but, in the case of childless couples, also upon proof of mutual consent (in exceptional circumstances divorce might even be granted where one partner claimed 'insurmountable aversion' against the other).

In reclaiming the sanctity of the Christian marriage against the permissive latitude of modern laws, the conservative jurists of the 1830s aligned themselves with the most reactionary groups among the Prussian aristocracy. In this context, the renewed emphasis on the double standard of adultery might appear as but a restoration of traditional assumptions about sexual morality. But the appearance of continuity is deceptive. If the success of the *Code Napoléon* had the effect of marginalising the revolutionary interlude of the *droit intermédiare*, the dominance of the Historical School of Law in nineteenth-century Germany gradually obliterated the achievements of the Enlightenment period. It was not before the reform of the divorce law in the 1970s that German legal thought re-established the connection with the ideas of that period. It was only then, and from the perspective of feminist legal history, that the reactive, specifically modern features of nineteenth-century patriarchal jurisprudence came to be fully recognised (Gerhard, 1978; Vogeli, 1988).

What was new in the arguments of Savigny – the founder of the Historical School and the most celebrated jurist of his time – was the attempt to ascertain the special normative structure of marriage within a system of private law premissed upon the principles of subjective will and individual freedom (Buchholz, 1979). Although it appeared in an altogether different philosophical framework this intention refers to a problem which we have already encountered in the debates on the Napoleonic code: for political reasons marriage had to be disconnected from the modern paradigm of contractual transactions that would justify divorce upon mutual consent. It had, on the other hand, to be rebuilt from principles which were compatible with the secular foundations of a modern legal system. Savigny's argument reconciled these conflicting demands by drawing on the distinction between contract and 'institution', on the one hand, and on a new language of sexual difference, on the other: while the regulation of matrimonial property was the proper domain of contractual freedom, the core of marriage, i.e. the personal relations between husband and wife, had to be derived from fundamentally different premises. To define marriage as an 'institution' was to claim for it the status of an ethical community, of an objective order independent of individual will and interest, and inaccessible to explanations in terms of formal rights and contractual obligations. Savigny identified the institution of marriage with three distinct purposes. With regard to the individual it had to be understood as the necessary form of a truly human existence; it guaranteed the ethical, non-contractual order of the state and, considered by its world historical significance, the 'elevated moral status of the whole female sex' (Savigny, 1850: 233, 271).

A normative conception of sexual difference written into the very definition of marriage was thus directly related to the purposes of the state. How closely, as a consequence, women's adultery became identified with the pathology of the political order can be gleaned from Savigny's endorsement of punishment. According to the existing law (i.e. the code of 1794), criminal charges for adultery could only be brought at the instigation of the innocent partner. The fact that legal practice seemed to make but little use of the punitive provisions of the law became a matter of increasing concern in those circles who sought to re-enforce the deterrent function of divorce proceedings. Debates on this issue focused on two questions – whether the state should punish adultery at all (rather than leave this task to the informal sanctions of religion and morality and to the penalties at the disposition of the civil law), and whether the punishment should be the same for both spouses (Savigny, 1845). In Savigny's account the two questions were inseparably linked. As the guardian of the public interest the state had to punish adultery just as it punished perjury. By the same token it was the wife's unfaithfulness that weighed more heavily in the scales of justice. Unlike her husband's deviance, her adultery 'violated the most vital interests of state, family and public morality alike' (Savigny, 1845: 451). Savigny's draft for a revision of the Prussian code would have sentenced women to imprisonment or incarceration for a period twice as long as that envisaged for men (Gerhard, 1978).

The demand for discriminatory punishment turned explicitly against the 'modern views on the position of women' (Savigny, 1845: 452) which had misled legislators in some countries to concede an equal obligation of conjugal fidelity. However, this 'reaction' did not base itself upon traditional beliefs in women's inferiority and the inherent frailty of their moral disposition. The double standard of adultery gained a new lease of legitimacy in perceptions of sexual difference – derived from Rousseau, Fichte and from the romantic celebration of diversity and polarity – which stressed the complementarity of male and female sexual character (Gerhard, 1978; Vogel, 1986): Because the 'elevated moral status of the female sex' was wholly enclosed in the inner sanctuary of conjugal love and fidelity any instance of sexual deviance on the part of a wife struck at the foundations of the marriage bond. Conversely, because a man, by nature destined for freedom, extended his activity into many spheres of life, his 'occasional lapse from virtue' could be understood as an isolated incident of no significant legal consequence. Her transgression was irredeemable, his could be forgiven and, indeed, such magnanimity would bestow nothing so much as honour and respect upon a wife (Savigny, 1845). Greater freedom thus corresponded to lesser responsibility. But this absurd perversion of moral principles was lost in the continuous reiteration of the assurance that the more exacting obligations and the punitive sanctions imposed on individual women were but so many expressions of the honour that the law accorded to the female sex as a whole.

Joined together, the shift from contract to 'institution' in the definition of marriage and a conception of sexual difference resonant with modern sensibilities effectively insulated the double standard of adultery against principles of individual right and formal equality. Within this normative framework the question of sexual property could not be raised. In a curious way a wife's obligation of fidelity did not even refer to rights held by her husband. It was claimed as if it were owed directly to the state.

Although it is thus concealed by a screen of higher political purposes, the partiality of the state to the husband's proprietary interests becomes transparent once we shift the focus of attention to the legal consequences of men's illicit sexual behaviour. How, in other words, was the law to attribute guilt and responsibility in relation to the offspring fathered by men outside marriage? The Prussian code had armed the unwed mother and her child with relatively generous claims against the father. The law compelled him to pay alimony and to provide for the expenses of pregnancy and confinement. Moreover, the woman of good repute was able to recover damages of up to one-fourth of the man's income. If she had been deceived by false promises of marriage, she was to be treated like a divorced wife. Most importantly, court procedures to establish paternity allowed her to raise claims against any one among several potential fathers of her child (Gerhard, 1978).

The revisionist projects of the 1840s and 1850s sought to retract these benefits which, in the view of Savigny, made the law an accomplice of 'adultery and fornication' (Buchholz, 1979: 321). They applauded the rigid prescriptions of the *Code Napoléon*, which had restored the barriers between the natural and the legal family temporarily levelled by the *droit intermédiaire*. The French Code not only revoked most of the illegitimate child's claims to sustenance and inheritance. The notorious article 340 ruled out any search and suit for paternity: *'La récherche de la paternité est interdite'*. The Prussian 'reformers' aimed at similar devices to insulate the bourgeois family against the consequences of men's sexual freedom. According to a decree enacted in 1854 the woman who had knowingly entertained a relationship with a married man had thereby forfeited all claims to compensation. The courts should not have the right to examine the moral record of a putative father. For 'where was the man steeled in the struggle against the adversities of life who might not be accused of some irregularity of this kind?' (Gerhard, 1978: 431). The female partners of such a man's vigorous educational escapades, on the other hand, had to submit to exacting tests of moral scrutiny. The rights of the unwed mother had to be asserted against the double barrier of the *exceptio plurium incumbentium* (intercourse with several men during the period of conception) and of evidence of good repute. Even worse, the claims of the child to alimony were no longer recognised independently (as in the code of 1794); they followed from the rights and, thus, from the moral reputation, of the mother.

The whole argument turned on the assumption that any leniency on the part of the law would be exploited, to the disadvantage of men, by the depraved members of the female sex. The sexual conduct and moral obligations of men themselves were not an issue. They did not count in the arbitrary construction of the 'public interest'. And the celebrated moral purity of the wife was but a thin veneer behind which the state and its law were free to force punitive measures upon all women who ended up on the wrong side of the divided standard of morality.

That the claimed political significance of women's adultery was an ideological construct and dependent upon particular interests and particular perceptions of the public good can be seen from the statement of an eighteenth-century Prussian civil servant who was involved in the preparation of the Civil Code of 1794. From a different perspective on the interests of the state the double standard of adultery might even be turned in the other direction:

As far as the interests of the state are concerned a wife's adultery cannot be judged as a graver offence than that of the husband. On the contrary, the former might even be less damaging, because the wife will give birth to legitimate children while the husband will produce illegitimate offspring, and, furthermore, because the seduction of a young woman by the husband is more disadvantageous to the state than the seduction of a young man by the wife.

(Gerhard, 1988: 420)

ADULTERY AND DIVORCE IN NINETEENTH-CENTURY ENGLAND: 'CONFUSION OF PROGENY CONSTITUTES THE ESSENCE OF THE CRIME'
(Dr Johnson, quoted in Thomas, 1959: 209)

In nineteenth-century England 'divorce meant adultery'; and adultery remained until not long ago the only legitimate ground upon which a marriage could be dissolved (Horstman, 1985: 4). The debates that surrounded the reform of the divorce laws in the period between 1840 and 1870 provide us with a model-case to explore the connections between the double standard of adultery, on the one hand, and the interests of property, on the other. Unlike France and Germany, however, England had experienced neither a political revolution nor the effects of a systematic reorganisation and codification of private law. It is thus more problematic to claim any significant changes in the normative framework in which the double standard was debated and justified.

By the middle of the century, England was the only Protestant country that had retained the Canon Law prohibitions against divorce. Only judicial separation, not divorce, could be obtained from the ecclesiastical courts. Although the church recognised adultery by either spouse as sufficient ground for a *separatio a mensa et thoro*, the prevailing laws of matrimonial property would have left most wives without the means of supporting themselves (Thomas, 1959). Upon obtaining a separation order from the church court a husband could then turn to the Common Law to sue the lover of his adulterous wife for trespass, assault and criminal conversation. The wife was not even a party to these transactions: she was herself the property the violation of which entitled the husband to file for damages (Horstman, 1985). Private Acts of Parliament could in exceptional circumstances grant a divorce. But the exorbitant costs of the procedures involved moved this remedy beyond the reach of all but the most wealthy and best-connected families. Moreover, out of the two hundred successful petitions recorded before 1857, only a handful were granted to women. A husband's adultery was deemed to have no legal relevance unless it was compounded by incest or bigamy. Those who sat in judgment over divorce cases were not unaware of the massive injustice to which the law was party. But here, too, the challenge brought against the double standard on grounds of individual claims to fair treatment tended to be defused by submitting the case to the superior imperatives of 'public morality' (Thomas, 1959)

The Matrimonial Causes Act of 1857 brought no sweeping changes (McGregor, 1957). By transferring jurisdiction over matrimonial matters to a secular court it extended the availability of divorce to the middle classes. It did not establish the equality of women and men in relation to adultery. While it added cruelty and desertion to the aggravating conditions on which a husband's adultery could be claimed against him, it preserved the old patterns of legal discrimination. When the Act passed through Parliament there was a general consensus that the sin committed by adultery was the same for both spouses but that different treatment stood justified by the significance of different consequences:

> A wife might without any loss of caste ... condone an act of adultery on the part of the husband; but a husband could not condone a similar act on the part of a wife. No one would venture that a husband could possibly do so, and for this, among other reasons ... that the adultery of the wife might be the means of palming suspicious offspring on the husband while the adultery of the husband could have no such effect with regard to the wife.
>
> (McGregor, 1957: 20)

In both substance and rhetoric the indictment of 'spurious issue' merely followed a tradition in which the presumption of certain paternity, understood as the bedrock of the social order, was the axiomatic reference point in all arguments about adultery. Does the tenacity of this presumption not suggest that the possessive claims at the core of the double standard are, indeed, rooted in a permanent, ahistorical constitution of male interests? Historians of Victorian England have drawn attention to the central function of the double standard in the moral orientations of the new middle classes manifest in a rigid code of 'Respectability' (Thomas, 1959; Horstman, 1985). Before the middle of the eighteenth century the threat of 'spurious issue' referred above all to the danger that estates and titles of the aristocracy might pass to bastards. This threat took on a new significance among the middle classes whose wealth was not tied up by the rules of primogeniture but transmitted by partible inheritance (Hoggett and Pearl, 1987). Only the most exacting demands on female chastity – and, conversely, the most austere sanctions imposed on adulterous wives – could, it seems, prevent the 'ultimate catastrophe' (Hoggett and Pearl, 1987: 401) that an imposter and false claimant of property might take his place at the heart of the family. The divorce law of 1857 took account of these interests and fears. The purpose of the reform was not to open avenues of easy divorce but to provide an effective deterrent both through the publicity of court trials and through the punitive measures that would follow upon adultery. The latter were aimed, in the first instance, at the adulterous wife who would lose her children as well as her property, and who in many cases would incur the double stigma of poverty and prostitution.

Similar evidence of a new, class-specific emphasis on the punitive functions of the adultery laws can be observed if, again, we consider the changes in the status of illegitimacy. The old Poor Law had charged both the mother and the reputed father of an illegitimate child with the duty of maintenance. Where 'fame of incontinence' was followed by punishment like public whipping, it would be imposed on both parents. The 'new' law of 1834 exempted the putative father from financial responsibilities and from the traditional criminal charges. The whole burden, moral and material, of illegitimacy was to fall on the mother. 'Just as the new poor law of 1834 presented a political triumph of philosophic radicalism by establishing an effective means of policing poverty, so it imposed middle-class morality upon pauper women by seeking to police their sexual virtue' (Hoggett and Pearl, 1987: 401). But rationalisations that appeared to focus exclusively on the functional necessity of preserving the order of property could not answer two obvious questions. Why were wives subjected to the double standard of punishment even where their adultery was not followed by the feared consequences, where there was neither 'confusion' nor 'progeny' (Thomas, 1959)? Second, if sexual fidelity was the necessary condition of security of property why should it, at least where normative principles were debated, not be made equally incumbent upon husbands as well as wives? What lay behind the legal enforcement of a differential sexual morality, as Thomas has compellingly argued, were men's proprietary claims not only on legitimate heirs but also, and independently, on women's bodies, i.e. their chastity. The exemption of men's infidelity from the stigma and sanctions of adultery could be maintained only at the cost of passing that stigma on to the 'spurious issue' fathered by them outside marriage. The 'bastard' – the child that the law imprisoned in an enclave of inferior status – rendered the consequences of men's adultery invisible.

CONCLUSION: THE BACKLASH OF PATRIARCHY

This chapter has examined the nature of property rights that sustained the double standard of adultery in nineteenth-century law and legal arguments. We have seen that in so far as they were overtly stated these rights were justified by the imperative of certain paternity. But the quest for absolute certainty of biological fatherhood could not explain why legislators and jurists of this period were concerned to reinforce the sheer physical power of restrictions which a divided standard of sexual morality imposed on women. The missing link in the chain of explanations and justifications must be sought in that other claim of ownership which remained largely concealed – in men's proprietary demands on women's sexuality. The focus on property rights has the advantage of stressing precisely those elements of power and coercion at the core of the adultery laws which are but inadequately captured if we consider the double standard merely in categories of prejudice, hypocrisy and other defects of moral judgement. The perspective on property does not allow us to forget that the presumption of the law which defined the status of a husband by a right of exclusive access to the wife's body while conceding to her lesser, conditional claims, was backed by the coercive power of the state. Women's unilateral obligation of sexual fidelity was created and sustained by force. It was enforced by the disabilities that they suffered in relation to divorce and, more tangibly, by the punitive sanctions of the criminal law.

However, property rights of this kind could in the nineteenth century no longer be claimed as personal rights. Under the constraints which derived from the individualist and contractual norms of modern private law the centre of legitimation shifted from men's private interests to those of the state. It was not, primarily, as a breach of contract (between private persons) that a wife's unfaithfulness was punished by the law. Rather, the husband's proprietary claims merged into, and became virtually undistinguishable from, the demands of the public order. The state itself appeared as the chief claimant on women's chastity.

I have argued that this shift of emphasis from the private to the public dimension of female adultery reflects the intentions of a *Patriarchalismus im Gegenstoss* (a 'backlash of patriarchy') (Gerhard, 1988: 466). Both the *droit intermédiaire* of the French Revolution and, in a different manner, the legal code of the Prussian paternalist state contained tendencies that pointed towards a single standard of conjugal obligations. The return to stricter enforcements of the double standard in the first half of the nineteenth century reveals the force of a political reaction which turned against the disorders associated with the French Revolution and, more generally, with the rationalist construction of authority in Enlightenment thought. Women's adultery, the focal point of disease in the pathology of marriage, served as a prism through which the perceived ills of modernity could be cast into sharp relief.

What was the reality to which such perceptions responded? It is impossible to tell whether this period witnessed any significant increase in the instances of women's adultery? What we do know is that there was much concern at the soaring divorce rate in the years that immediately followed on the legalisation of divorce (i.e. in France after 1792, in England after 1857, in Prussia in the first decades of the nineteenth century), and that this concern was prompted particularly by the unexpected number of women who sought to escape from their marriages (Sagnac, 1898; Phillips, 1980; Horstman, 1985). The salient point is, however, that such observations, whether well-founded or not, were placed in a nexus of negative meanings that directly linked instances of women's freedom to the breakdown of the social order. This general tendency emerges with particular clarity in the vilification of those women-turned-men who joined the struggle in the streets of revolutionary Paris (Vogel, 1990), in the hysteria that greeted the 'emancipation of the flesh' postulated by the Saint Simonians

(Horstman, 1985; Schnapper, 1987), in the apprehensions at the surge of mass poverty that dominated the debates on sexual deviance in England (Hoggett and Pearl, 1987). What these examples have in common is the determination to devolve responsibility for the general crisis of modern society and for the uncertainties of an uncharted future to women's sexual morality.

The intention to tighten the disciplinary power of the law over women's bodies might typically present itself as a return to older traditions of confirmed sanctity which had but temporarily been suspended by the subversive spirit of the modern age. Such legitimations might call upon the universal consensus of all civilised nations, on the enduring authority of the Roman law, on the moral superiority of the female sex since the advent of the Christian religion, or simply on the unbroken continuity of ancient customs. But whatever tradition was thus claimed on behalf of the double standard of adultery, it was a tradition *invented* for specific political purposes. In obscuring their own origins as a reaction against alternative, more egalitarian conceptions of marriage, the dominant languages of nineteenth-century legal thought created a powerful myth of historical continuity. This myth distorted the disruptions and discontinuities in the history of patriarchal law and silenced the memory of the emancipatory potential that might have developed from them.

Chapter 8

Mothers as citizens
Feminism, evolutionary theory and the reform
of Dutch family law 1870–1910

Selma Sevenhuijsen

INTRODUCTION

Although the social and political status of women has been
discussed within political theory over a long period of time (Coole,
1988), the end of the nineteenth century is a crucial period for the
emergence of concepts of female/feminist citizenship. Feminism
developed in a politico-legal culture within which concepts of
'woman', 'politics' and 'rights' could not really be linked. Women
were supposed to be the inhabitants of civil society living under
the governance of fathers and husbands, and not active citizens of
political society. Citizenship was a male condition, an identity which
men of the possessing classes could claim as owners of property
and as fathers of families. The emergence of a broadly based politically
oriented women's movement, aiming at the conquest of legal and
political rights produced a substantial debate on the gender-basis
of rights, in fields where legal and political theory had previously
spoken in the seemingly gender-neutral language of 'individuals'.

In this chapter I argue that the study of family law reform is
crucial for understanding the emergence of women's citizenship.
The non-citizenship of women was established in legal discourse
around family law, against which feminism waged its criticism. The
point I want to make, is that it was not only categories of 'rights'
that were at stake in the debate connected to the reform of family
law, but categories of 'woman' as well. There was no clear-cut or
fixed identity of 'woman', that could be claimed to be the possessor
of 'rights', precisely because 'rights' were so heavily moulded in
favour of male needs and identities.

The newly emerging debates about women's rights were thus
also debates about the conditions under which women were to be

admitted to the legal and political order of the state, and about the conditions of their exclusion. Images of motherhood, sexual identity and women's economic position were all contested. In a more extensive study about the reform of Dutch family law at the end of the nineteenth century I have analysed these discourses from the perspective of the political debates on unmarried motherhood (Sevenhuijsen, 1987).[1] When the needs of illegitimate children and unmarried mothers became a political issue, the leading legal presumptions about marriage and patriarchal fatherhood became more and more strained. Here I will concentrate on the impact of evolutionary theory in this discursive field. Between 1890 and 1900 a broad range of participants on the debate on family law framed their arguments within its terms.

In the first section I shall give a brief and necessarily schematic overview of the central rules concerning motherhood and fatherhood in nineteenth-century Dutch family law. In the second, I provide a sketch of the political backgrounds against which issues concerning women's rights in family law were becoming a subject of feminist concern. In the third, I shall concentrate on the different versions of evolutionary theory which became influential in this discursive field in the 1890s.

NINETEENTH-CENTURY FAMILY LAW AND WOMEN'S EXCLUSION FROM CITIZENSHIP

The prototype of the legal subject in nineteenth-century law was the enlightened male individual, in the possession of a certain amount of property and the rationality required to recognise his interests and govern his family. Liberal political theory conceived of political society as a community of male property owners who were at the same time heads of households. Men governed their families and came together in the political community to serve their wider interests. As fathers, men were supposed to transmit property, skills and traditions to their male heirs. Kinship rules which regulated marriage, legitimacy and illegitimacy can be said to have been aimed at guaranteeing the blood-tie between father and son, which derived its meaning from this male social function. It was legal marriage that constructed patriarchal fatherhood. Although nineteenth-century Dutch family law cannot be characterised as a 'classical' patriarchal system, in the sense of

Roman Law in which fathers govern larger families until their death, it was clearly patriarchal in a sense that nuclear families were headed by fathers, unrestricted by any rights of women as mothers or by potential interventions by the state. In the Civil Code of 1838 (which was virtually copied from the French *Code civil* that was imported into Holland in 1810) certain rules concerning the legal construction of fatherhood were introduced which deviated from old Dutch Law before the French Revolution. The two guiding rules on marriage remained the same, namely the rule of 'marital power', which stated that the husband is the head of the family, and the rule of *pater est quem nuptiae demonstrant* (the husband is assumed to be the father of the child).

The main changes concerned the position of unmarried mothers. Whereas old Dutch Law acknowledged the rule *mater semper certa est*, this rule was now abolished and traditional avenues for suits concerning the paternity of children born out wedlock were abolished as well. An unmarried mother could have a legal family tie with her child but only if she had established a legal 'recognition'. She could do this either voluntarily, or under a legal order. A man could establish a legal recognition as well, but in his case only on a voluntary basis. For this legal process he needed the permission of the mother. If both parents had recognised a child, the man exercised paternal power. If only the woman had established legal recognition it was in a sense unclear whether she exercised paternal power or whether the child was under her custody. So whether married or unmarried, women were not bearers of 'automatic' rights as mothers. Marriage was an institution that created fatherhood as a structuring element in gender relations, which was laid down in a set of rights and in a lesser sense in duties concerning women and children. The legal rules on the recognition of children born out of wedlock were mainly constructed as an 'entry' to the full legitimation of children through a successive marriage: legal recognition was supposed to be a proof of biological truth.

Women hardly figured in this legal system. They lived under the legal governance of either fathers or husbands. Only when they remained unmarried, did they have the legal capacity to perform some legal acts in the sphere of private law on their own. This non-citizenship of women could be defended along several lines (if it was necessary to defend it at all). Women were not supposed to be in the possession of reason, or to be incapable of committing legal acts, or they were supposed to have consented to this legal construction. Besides this, it was argued that women derived protection and rights to maintenance from this social and legal system which was necessary for their natural destiny as mothers.

There were, however, some other, more marginal identities in which women figured in this legal system, and in the intellectual landscape of male legal theorists. In the first place she could be an adulterous wife, in which case she was treated differentially compared to the adulterous husband. Adultery for a wife was a punishable act in penal law, for a husband it was not. The legal rationale for this different treatment was the possibility of women becoming pregnant and bringing 'strange' blood into the family: a consequence of the dominance of patriarchal kinship motives in law. In family law adultery was for both partners a ground for divorce.

In the second place, women figured as seducers. The main presumptions about unmarried mothers were that they were intentional seducers of men, conspiring to gain wealth by becoming pregnant and bringing legal claims to family capital. For this reason it was considered dangerous to give women the legal possibility of bringing a paternity suit. Responsible men were supposed to take care of their illegitimate offspring of their own free will. In this, as in other respects, the enlightened male individual was the prototype of law, or perhaps it is better to say that his existence was a crucial legal fiction. This can be seen in the sharp lines drawn in legal discourse between 'legal duties' and 'moral duties'.

We can conclude that women were largely absent in nineteenth-century family law and in the domain of active citizenship. They were absent in the sense of being legal subjects and bearers of legally enforceable rights. Mothers were supposed to be willingly under the governance of husbands. Where women were present, this was often in connection with sexuality, which was presented as a danger to the social order. Law produced a legal discourse in which woman's reproductive potential and her sexuality were central to her identity, and in which hierarchy was supposed to be the normal state of affairs between the sexes. Motives of kinship and property were dominant in this respect: sexual considerations were subsidiary to these. In both respects, as a mother and as a sexual being women were conceptualised as persons who should not be permitted to enter the legal order in their own right. When demanding female entrance to this legal order, feminism had to confront these rigid constructions of womanhood.

The emergence of critical approaches to the legal order

Between 1870 and 1890, on the eve of the emergence of organised feminism, several movements for social and moral reform formulated a range of new issues for which legal reform was deemed necessary. Reform-oriented liberals, worried about poverty and criminality, designed new proposals for population policies in which early marriage and the regulation of family size came to be viewed positively. Their views encompassed proposals for the liberalisation of divorce and more rights for women within marriage. In the more restrictive versions of social liberalism, children figured as future criminals and prostitutes, driven towards this fate by poverty and lack of paternal supervision and authority. From 1878, fundamentalist Protestants waged anti-prostitution campaigns that were gradually broadened to include proposals for paternity suits and for moral reform of marital relations. Social liberals and Protestant reformers worked together in designing child-protection policies in which the position of illegitimate children was problematised. Their policies clashed, however, on issues connected to birth control, moral reform and the legal position of married women. Between 1880 and 1900 proposals for restriction and liberalisation of divorce were in conflict. This led to a political stalemate around divorce that lasted until 1970, when divorce on the grounds of irretrievable break-down and mutual consent was finally allowed.

Although there was at the end of the nineteenth century a wide variety of views and reform proposals, one can say that the conflicts about legal reform concentrated in many respects on the general direction of change that should be taken. On the one hand there was a radical approach, connected to radical liberalism, free-thinkers and to a lesser extent to early socialism. It argued that the main principles of family law had to be changed, and presented a clear view of new guiding principles. Equality of rights, responsibilities and duties inside and outside marriage were the main goals in this radical approach. This implied that in effect the 'function' or dominant meaning of marriage as a medium of patriarchal fatherhood would be undermined, although mostly not intentionally. Differences in the sexual and parental identities of men and women remained important in this approach, they were not, however, considered to be a legitimate argument for differences in legal treatment and rights between men and women. In this respect the argument put forward by John Stuart Mill (whose book *The Subjection of Women* was translated into Dutch in 1870) that gendered characteristics were 'produced' by inhibitions on the freedom of women, were highly influential among progressive Dutch political thinkers (Mill, 1869; Jansz, 1990).

In the second approach, associated with moderate or 'social' liberalism and Protestant moral reform movements, a whole range of social problems like poverty, prostitution, infanticide, criminality and alcoholism were put forward for which existing legal arrangements had no solution, or which were even in some respects supposed to be generated by existing law. In this approach legal marriage, with the husband as head of household was to remain the core of society, politics and family law. The harmful effects of these hierarchical relations could, it was argued, be countered in a piecemeal way by reforms in the direction of more justice and greater equality in moral judgements.

When organised feminism emerged, it had to handle this tension between radical and moderate reform as well. The founding of the first autonomous women's organisation Vrije Vrouwen Vereeniging (Free Women's League) in 1889 and the publication of the related journal *Evolutie*, starting in 1893, played a prominent role in the proliferation of discussions about the direction of change. *Evolutie* set the tone for this debate by outlining in its first issues a rudimentary programme of equality between men and women. In its demands for equal education and labour-market participation, for equal political rights and equal rights within family law, a radical democratic programme for gender politics and female citizenship was formulated. In this programme the borderline between marriage and non-marriage was becoming vague. Men and women were to become citizens as persons in their own right, being equal by birth. Autonomy, respect and love were to take the place of hierarchy, exploitation and marriage of convenience. This 'programme' was connected to a critique of sexual difference which fits within the tradition of John Stuart Mill. Against theorists who stated that women were by nature submissive, docile or vain, the standard answer was brought forward that social structures and legal arrangements had 'forced' them to become that way. The doctrine of sexual difference was exposed as a device to keep women in their position of subordination.

In the broader women's movement there was no consensus about this radical democratic conception of sexual politics. In the course of the ensuing debate several positions on the reform of family law were articulated, in which the above-mentioned tension between radical and moderate reform can be recognised. This debate can be interpreted as a discursive terrain in which concepts of motherhood, equality, autonomy and the basis of female citizenship were constructed, contested and proliferated.

The first position, to be characterised as *equality*, was voiced by Wilhelmina Drucker, the chief editor of *Evolutie*. Under the title 'Fatherhood and motherhood' she published six articles, which set the tone of the debate (Drucker, 1895). The social and political regulation of parenthood was a central element in her social theory. She saw the history of mankind as being divided in two phases: matriarchy and patriarchy. The first was based on the familial and the political power of the mother. Some tribes still lived in this phase, in which a 'female lust for power' reigned. Patriarchy was characterised by male power in the family and the public sphere based on the ownership of land, women and children. On this basis a sexual division of labour had developed in which women did the work around the house and men concentrated on political power, warfare and religion. Religion was an institution of patriarchal power which had to be replaced by the rational and enlightened knowledge of modern science.

This schematic conception of history was clearly a moral diagnosis, it served Drucker to design a moral vision of future society and a criterion to judge different strategies. Both matriarchy and patriarchy were seen by her as 'unnatural', and based on power and usurpation. Nature was still buried under power, but it had to be the guideline for a society of the future. For Drucker, this implied that the principle that everybody was born equal had to be the starting point. The natural family, based on the ties of blood, ovum and semen, was to be taken as the norm: family law had to be structured around this principle. There was no reason to benefit either the father or the mother. She labelled future society as 'parental duty'. This meant that the state should form a system of detailed prescription, supervision and punishment around the responsibilities and rights of parenthood.

With her articles, Drucker explicitly attacked a small and incoherent group of women, who were representatives of a second position within the feminist spectrum. Their position can be characterised as one of *autonomy*. Within this position a subdivision can be made between women who spoke in terms of oppression and women who spoke in terms of sexual difference. Both used rudimentary concepts of mother right in a positive form. The oppression argument emerged in the context of political campaigns against the prohibition of paternity suits. Against the dominant feminist attitude some women took the position that maintenance duty by fathers should not be made obligatory, because it was a humiliation for a woman if she had to accept support from the man who had seduced her, or if she had to accept a forced marriage. It was thought better to wage a struggle for mother right and to eliminate the difference between legitimate and illegitimate children. The state was to be required to take responsibility for the education and maintenance of all children. Public responsibility was to be an alternative to slavery. So concepts of autonomous motherhood and a strong social state went hand in hand.

The difference argument transcended the imagery of the fallen woman, and started from a plea for sexual autonomy for women in general. It judged sexual abstinence for women as acceptable if it was freely chosen, but it was not to be seen as the only natural way of behaviour, as many feminists stated. The only 'natural' thing was that women were by their reproductive capacity the most capable of raising children, and that women were accordingly monogamous by nature. Men were not supposed to be monogamous, because the link between love and sexuality was looser in their case. In future society women should be able to be autonomous in economic and social respects, so that they could have a relationship with the man they loved and could stop this when love had faded. Because women were monogamous, there would be no risk that paternity was uncertain: in this respect legal arrangements were deemed superfluous.

The third position, which was influenced by social-liberalism as well as by Protestant ideas of moral reform, can be characterised as a *social-problem* approach. It was by far the most influential within the women's movement. In this approach marriage was to be reformed to become a true union of love. Sexual difference was seen as natural: women and men had different dispositions and identities. Psychological characteristics could not be reduced to social circumstances. Instead, legal and social arrangements had to be forged in such a way that natural difference could be effective for social relations based on justice. The unity between male and female could bring harmony in social and political affairs.

This position implied no clear-cut conception of how legal rights should be framed. It could lead to proposals for moderate change under the argument that men had a natural propensity for leadership, hence women should claim only subsidiary rights. It could also lead to more radical proposals for equal rights in family law or in politics. Proposals for legal reform were in general designed more in connection with concepts of protection, moral reform and the solution of 'social problems', than in connection with legal equality.

Unmarried motherhood was one of these social problems, and the doctrine of the critique of the dual standard of morality was used as a way of diagnosing it.[2] Poverty, seduction, prostitution and criminality all remained important sources of complaint. The fallen woman was the prototype of the unmarried mother. The borderline between her and the decent woman, as well as between marriage and illegitimacy, had to be firmly watched. Female solidarity, professional help and legal provisions were to give shape to a public responsibility for the destitution of the unmarried mother. A more direct responsibility by the state, as proposed in the first two positions, was dismissed by the argument that it undermined the family, marriage and the responsibility of biological parents. The introduction of automatic parental rights for unmarried mothers was not urgent in this programme. At its best the introduction of these rights was favoured because it made legal liability clearer in cases where children were to be removed from parental control and placed under the supervision of child protection agencies.

We can conclude that within the women's movement as well as in broader political currents as described above, the debate on gender politics and women's rights and citizenship circled around a range of issues and questions in connection with sexual difference, monogamy, love, the regulation of sexuality, the meaning of marriage and the meaning of motherhood and fatherhood. These issues were discussed on a more general level within the debate on evolution, patriarchy and mother right, which had already been going on for several decades (Coward, 1983). Evolutionary theory was a crucial intellectual stage on which the 'Woman's Question' was fought out around the turn of the century.

THE IMPACT OF EVOLUTIONARY THEORY: THE STRUGGLE BETWEEN TWO MODELS

Although Darwinism gave a strong impetus to theorising about the development of human societies in broad historical periodisations, it is important to remember that this way of theorising emerged against the background of an older tradition in social and political theory. This older tradition saw the development of state and society in terms of stages in history. The reception of Darwin's work marked a point in this intellectual development where biological concepts began to occupy a more central position in social theory and political strategies.

The origins of this intellectual scheme are traceable in the emergence of liberal contract theory and the debate on natural law. The status of patriarchalism and the authority of the father was one of the issues in this debate (Brennan and Pateman, 1979). Classical patriarchalism stated that the authority of the father stood at the origin of society. Political authority of the king was a continuation of the authority of the father, and duty of obedience to these authorities rested on the same grounds. In opposition to this view, liberal contract theory claimed the existence of a society of free individuals. To state the legitimacy of equal citizenship and of central political authority, the analogy between the authority of the father and the authority of the king had to be broken down.

In the work of John Locke this endeavour is an important element (Locke, 1690; see Locke, 1967). In the state of nature everybody was born equal. On the other hand, he stated that there was a natural division of labour between the sexes, emerging from the fact that women were pregnant for a large part of their lives. As a consequence, women needed protection from men. The social contract was, in his view, agreed upon by male heads of households. Men exercised political rights because they were 'abler and stronger'. Although women were persons in their own right, they consented to this situation by entering into the marriage contract. In Locke's work, citizenship was linked to property in a broad sense. Ownership had a meaning for family relations and male identity and rights as well. Men should have the right to pass their property on to their favourite sons, and this right should have priority over the right of governments to claim property.

The 'state of nature' was, in Locke's theory, a speculation about the historical existence of social relations prior to the conclusion of the political contract. In the work of John Hobbes it amounted more to a series of deductive statements about human psychology (Hobbes, 1651). The state of nature was, in his conception, characterised by the reign of passions instead of reason. This led to the threat of a general war. Civilisation, art and production emerged when man transferred his rights and freedoms to the sovereign, who guaranteed property and peace. 'Nature' implied that children were under the governance of women, because paternity was never certain. The establishment of paternal authority was based on the need for protection. Within marriage a woman placed herself and her children under the protection of family heads. This implies that the family was not based on nature, blood-ties, or 'natural' responsibilities of parents, but on power and contract.

Liberal political theory was thus confronted with a dilemma about the relation between the origin of society, political authority, the family and gender relations. Was the family, conceived as a hierarchical relation between man, woman and children based on biological ties and 'natural' identities or was it primarily a political and legal construction? In this dilemma we can recognise questions about the function of the law in the construction of fatherhood. It is remarkable that this question was so strongly framed and answered in terms of origins of society and the connection to the sovereign power of the state.

In eighteenth-century political theory the scheme of two stages was developed further in the context of contract theory and speculations about the origins of society. Representations about newly discovered tribes now played an important part in speculating about the state of nature (Meek, 1976; Stein, 1980). Different schemes were proposed in which sex, love and property were combined in a variety of ways. Adam Smith connected the stages of history to a fixed sequence of four modes of production (hunting, grazing, agriculture and commerce). In the work of the Scottish philosopher John Millar, these stages were connected to the development of marriage, parenthood and sexual customs. For his description of the state of nature Millar drew on travel records about so-called 'primitive' people who lived, according to his observations, in a state of sexual promiscuity. He was one of the first authors who spoke in terms of a primitive matriarchy that had taken place during the hunting phase of production. Agriculture introduced monogamous patriarchal marriage. For women this was a progressive moment, because love, respect and steadiness took the place of wild passion and licentiousness.

The importance of these ideas of 'conjectural history' is that they contained an area of speculation about the natural in which women, gender identity and the family took a prominent place. The question about the origin of the family was connected to discourses in which all kinds of psychological characteristics were ascribed, in a dichotomous way, to 'male' and 'female'. The relationship between passion, nature, reason and interest was debated in this context (Rendall, 1987). The relation between these phenomena was placed in an evolutionary scheme, a way of thinking in large time spans, which contained speculations about the past as well as the future. In the second half of the nineteenth century this way of theorising about society became a central paradigm in social theory (Burrow, 1970; Coward, 1983).

Around 1860 the debate took a new turn following from publications within the discipline of historical jurisprudence. Bachofen (1861) introduced the idea that prior to patriarchal society, mother-right societies had existed where kinship was dominated by ties with the mother, and women had a dominant political position. Matriarchy was preceded by a stage of primitive promiscuity. Mother right was in his view equivalent to nature, irrationality and religion. The bond between child and father was based on distance, rationality and knowledge. The triumph over mother right was a triumph of reason over passion; the love of the father had created a bond between family, the nation and the state.

In the same period the English legal theorist, Maine, stated that patriarchal family clans were the original social form (Maine, 1861). The authority of the father was based on legal power, the *patria potestas*, and had no connection with biology, blood-ties or nature. Thus, the dilemma of 'nature' versus 'legal power' remained a dominant issue in speculations about the origins of society. The position of the father and the meaning of fatherhood was at the heart of the arguments in this field.

In this context, Darwin published in 1871 his work on the descent of man (Darwin, 1871). His contribution was an important step towards a firm statement of the naturalness of the biological family and male dominance. By comparing man with other primates he repudiated the idea of primitive promiscuity, and replaced it by an idea of original polygamy. The strongest men were able to appropriate the most beautiful women. In females this characteristic was more advanced because it was important in their selection. In the next stage, monogamy came about. This was not harmful to women because they could manipulate their beauty. Men were by nature more aggressive than women. Natural instincts led towards monogamy, phenomena like infanticide, early marriages and polyandry were adjustments to unnatural situations.

To understand the impact of late-nineteenth-century Darwinism on the debate on women's citizenship we should distinguish between roughly two versions of evolutionary theory, which combatted each other continuously in the 1880s and 1890s. The first is a progressively minded, socialist evolution version, and the second is a conservative-liberal one.

Socialist evolutionary theory is most clearly and coherently stated by Bebel in his classical work *Women under Socialism*, that was widely read among early socialists and feminists in the Netherlands (Bebel, 1897). Bebel tried to combine Darwin, Marx, Bachofen and Morgan in what can be called a design of a socialist moral politics. From Darwin he borrowed the idea of selection, the struggle for existence and the survival of the fittest, which he combined with a marxian view of class struggle. But he criticised Darwin and his followers for stating that this development was analogous for humans and animals. The difference between animals and humans was that man was in the possession of reason. The importance of reason was that it enabled mankind to know the development of society and could thus lead towards a higher stage of civilisation. From Bachofen and Morgan, he borrowed the idea of the original stage of mother-right societies. Western civilisation had developed from a combination of patriarchal power, the introduction of private property and the oppression of women within monogamous marriage. Phenomena like prostitution, infanticide, illegitimacy and abortion were all consequences of the vicious system of private property and the connected male urge for possession. This meant that, contrary to the dominant ideas on evolution, monogamy and the development of social relations were not progressive at all for women: it had meant the loss of freedom and integrity.

In future society, marriage would be founded on true sexual love. Natural sexual instincts should be freed and women would be emancipated from sexual slavery. The suppression of sexual instincts was a source of malaise in both sexes and was a curb to the healthy influence of nature. As a consequence, several forms of 'unnatural satisfaction' existed, which went hand in hand with unhealthy circumstances in the workplace and the home. True parental love and marriage based on love were only possible in a socialist society, characterised by communism and communal property. When private property was abolished, inheritance rights would no longer dominate the arrangement of marriage and the relations between the sexes. Women would be able to choose their own work, to contract a marriage from free will and to terminate it when love had vanished. By the granting of freedom and equality to women the ideas of the French Revolution would be completed.

Bebel connected this positive ideal of freedom for women to a concept of matriarchy, a return to social circumstances which were, in his view, by far the most favourable for women. Matriarchy was characterised by female activity and equality. Matriarchy of the future was a higher stage in civilisation, however, because the pernicious struggle between the sexes would be replaced by harmonious co-operation and love.

The conservative–liberal version of evolutionary theory was influenced by Darwin as well, but in a much more sociobiological and pessimistic vein than the socialist one. In the work of the Dutch sociologist Wijnaendts Francken, we can see a mixture of several influences from biology, legal theory and ethnology, combined with the moral politics of social liberalism. His work is important because it marks a point in academic evolutionary theory in which the 'Woman Question' was redefined by the emergence of modern *political* feminism. The importance of sexual difference was the main point that worried him. His explicit aim was to develop a sociological theory about marriage in which biology played the prominent role.

In his first book on this subject, the 'facts' of reproduction and impregnation were his starting point (Wijnaendts Francken, 1894). Natural evolution had brought a sexual division of labour between the active male and the passive female. Man was characterised by force and exposure to danger, woman needed protection to fulfil her natural reproductive functions. This implied that women selected lovers who were physically strong and could protect them and their children. Sexual instinct united the sexes with the aim of the preservation of the species. Male sexual instinct was larger and more diffuse, female instinct was directed towards reproduction.

Marriage, however, was primarily a *social* institution, connected to the introduction of private property. After a stage of original matriarchy, women had become the property of men. He did not, however, connect matriarchy to a concept of 'mother right'. Wijnaendts Francken preferred the dominant ethnological thesis of his time, namely that motherly kinship and matrilocality existed, but gynocracy was a myth. Male dominance in the family and in larger society was considered universal. When marriage had become the norm, the husband began to consider her children as his. This implied that the original bond between men and children was not based on biology, but on marriage. When man had got knowledge of his contribution to biological reproduction, he acquired the wish to inherit his property to his biological posterity: monogamy was born. The duty of maintenance was important, because it prevented polygamy.

Although Wijnaendts Francken made, just as Bebel did, a connection between monogamy and private property, this did not have a negative connotation. Instead, he saw property, fatherhood and monogamy as essential organisational principles of society. And in contrast to Bebel, he voiced uncertainty about the last phase of evolutionary development. Monogamy was in his opinion by far the most developed stage of civilisation, and the most favourable for women. Under monogamy equality and the elevation of women were the norm, and women could derive rights from their position within marriage. He depicted free love as the opposite of monogamy. Free love was detrimental to women and children because parental love did not count, while the passions of sexual love were too overwhelming. Marriage should be reformed in the direction of affection. Accordingly the numerical relation between the sexes and the selection process of partners had to be reformed. In this way abuses like prostitution and unmarried motherhood could be prevented. Procreation had to be limited, and paternity suits had to be introduced as a preventive measure against crime, prostitution and poverty.

Accordingly, the Woman Question was to be defined as a marriage question. By better education and by early marriages, natural relations could take the lead. Celibacy and the delay of marriage were unnatural. For men because they had a natural longing for a home of their own, with women and children; for women because their nature was characterised by love, sacrifice and the need for guidance. Women were, in his eyes, conservative and could not be creative. If women could not satisfy their natural needs, they would look for unnatural surrogates like sport, eccentricity and emancipation. The women's movement was a danger for society when it strived after an unnatural erosion of sexual difference.

Within 4 years after the publication of *The Evolution of Marriage* (1894) Wijnaendts Francken and other writers sharpened the normative element of this version of evolutionary theory. Sexual difference came to the forefront as a natural element of society, and accordingly, ideals about equality formed the main target of criticism.

In an article in 1896 Wijnaendts Francken argued for the importance of sexual difference on the basis of the work of Herbert Spencer, who had stated that social differentiation was the leading element of the evolutionary process (Wijnaendts Francken, 1896). Wijnaendts Francken attacked the statement of John Stuart Mill that differences in sexual character had evolved as a response to social circumstances, and turned this relationship around: society was formed on the basis of sexed characteristics. In relation to some characteristics women scored higher than men: self-sacrifice, altruism and moral elasticity. But next to this he ascribed to women a list of characteristics, which meant that they needed male guidance. He mentioned, for example, revengefulness and coquetry, but stressed characteristics in relation to intellectuality and reason. Women were seldom honest, they lacked love of the truth; they had an inclination towards exaggeration, were less objective and partial in their judgement. They lacked the capability of abstract reason and philosophy, and seldom reflected for long periods, etc. He considered these differences affirmed by anatomical research on the size of the skull. The conclusion was that women were definitely different, but not more or less worthy than men: they were equivalent to men. Men and women were supposed to complement each other within marriage, under male guidance of course. Unmarried women were malicious and bitter, a 'third sex'. And again he criticised political reforms: the border-lines between 'woman', 'rights' and 'politics' remained firmly drawn.

It is precisely this element of female political identity that was shifted by the publications on the woman question by one of the founding fathers of Dutch sociology S.R. Steinmetz in 1895–6 (Steinmetz, 1895; 1896). He was educated in the same academic circles as Wijnaendts Francken. His articles contained a plea for scientific knowledge about women, which he characterised as a modern positive science that had to replace common sense about women and socialist and neo-Malthusian ideologies as well. Sociology had to construct a 'positive technique' or 'socio-technique', where religion, natural law, and reason had failed. Social-Darwinism, sociobiology and eugenics were combined in a discourse that took sexual difference and the sexual division of labour as its point of departure.

Men were, according to Steinmetz, characterised by aggression and warfare, women by reproductive tasks. Women's productive labour was an 'aberration' from evolution. Future society should be based on peace and freedom, and the natural laws of division of labour would accordingly take the lead again. Private property, the biological family, the interdependence of motherhood and fatherhood were to serve as guiding principles. 'Happiness' meant that women should devote themselves to domestic labour.

A specific concept of love took a central position in Steimetz's work. He deemed true altruistic love possible only on the basis of difference, and not on the basis of comradeship as Mill had argued. He, too, accused feminism of tending towards 'unisexuality' and accordingly, to the abolition of love and the family. Not equality, but the family with the mother at its centre, should be the end-point of evolution. It was the aim of science to design a strategy that was as much as possible in accordance with the desirable last phase of evolution. It was the mutual dependence of mother and father that made the family a real family. If this principle was not understood, male polygamy would return. Promoting female independence and freedom implied that women would lose because of the naturally dissolute behaviour of men. But the biggest problem of all was that fatherhood was than doomed to decay.

Unmarried motherhood was, in Steinmetz's conception, following the then common anthropological wisdom, a 'matriarchal survival', that had to be abolished on the way to 'parental right' as the last stage of evolution. The programme for family-law reform had to be founded on the desirability of social differentiation. At this point Steinmetz constructed a negative mirror image of feminism, which was, according to him, based on 'divorce with mutual consent, free love and mother-right'. These phenomena were in his view the inevitable consequence of the principal of equal rights within marriage. Instead of autonomy and independence, protection and dependence should be taken as the leading principles. Man was the natural leader of the family, natural women consented in this state of affairs, and if women did not consent, nobody should care. It is clear that 'mother-right' or 'matriarchy' served as a negative image. The course of evolution, which was once judged to be progressive and positive, was not so certain any more. If official policies were not framed in the right way, mankind would fall back into matriarchy.

Family law, according to Steinmetz, should be reformed along the following lines: community of property between the spouses, more parental rights for the married mother and guarantees for women against abuse by men. Men who neglected their obligations should be heavily punished. Divorce was to be an instrument to mould the family in desirable directions which implied that specifications should be made for the grounds of divorce. Family law should thus be seen as *public* law. In his scheme this meant that it was to be an instrument in a state-guided construction of gender and sexual difference. Women were to be admitted to the legal order, on the strict condition that they remained loving mothers under the guidance of husbands.

The public aspects of women's citizenship were designed in a similar mode. While Wijnaendts Francken had disapproved of female political activities and labelled this as a 'surrogate' for their natural inclinations, Steinmetz allowed women a political identity *as mother*. This new 'Ideal Woman' had to be the leader of all women. As a mother, woman had moral qualities, that could counteract male aggression and warfare. Man would become peaceful if he could find happiness in his family. As a mother, woman could do a great amount of useful social labour, and should even get the vote. Motherly interests could be promoted. But one should watch carefully in case it was the other female species, the unmarried spinster, who took the lead. Under her direction society would be contaminated by unfeminine influences. But because patriarchy was over, her interests were not protected by the family. Instead, the state had to protect her, in order to prevent social contamination.

CONCLUSIONS

For contemporary observers it is very tempting to depict both Wijnaendts Francken and Steinmetz as anti-feminists. This observation can, next to their explicit anti-feminist statements, be supported by reference to attacks on their views in the feminist press, headed by Wilhelmina Drucker in *Evolutie*. As an overall conclusion this would be misleading, however, for the very reason that the meaning of sexual difference in the construction of female citizenship was contested within feminism as well. Connected to this we must appreciate that the meaning of 'feminism' was not fixed either: there was a wide variety of opinions about the directions the women's movement should take and about the 'ideal society' that should be the point of reference.

The opinions of both authors reflect an area of disagreement among the ranks of those who considered themselves as involved with feminism. There was, for example, disagreement about the question of whether married women or their unmarried sisters should get the vote first, because suffrage for unmarried women fitted more easily in the legal arrangements concerning electoral eligibility. This question was connected to the problem of sequence: should women strive after citizenship in the sphere of private law, before getting an equal status as political citizens, or should this happen the other way around? And next to this, it was connected to the role of single women within the women's movement.

With respect to the issue of education, the attitude of Steinmetz and Wijnaendts Francken can be convincingly labelled as anti-feminist: most feminists agreed on the desirability of equal entrance to the educational system for women. In respect to the goals of education, however, opinions differed. For example, was education a prerequisite for economic independence and autonomous womanhood, or for being better wives and mothers?

The impact of the conservative version of evolutionary theory can be best evaluated in the arguments around the meaning of sexual difference and the meaning of law and legal arrangements. Woman was shaped in its discourse as the mirror and opposite of man, and as a person who is by nature inclined to subservience. By this argument, political rights and autonomous agency could be ascribed to her in a minimal way, and on strict conditions. Law, legal reform and the definition of female citizenship were judged to be instrumental in defining 'woman'. The normal woman was designed as mother and wife: competing identities were categorised and marginalised. The borderlines between the decent, married woman, the sexual woman and the unmarried mother had to be clearly watched. The emergence of the women's movement had added a potential identity to this enumeration which threatened to blur the distinctions between motherly and sexual identities of women: the free woman. Negative utopias about the disintegration of society and civilisation when women would be accorded rights as mothers can be interpreted as an expression of substantial cultural fears about the autonomy of women.

The issue of rights of unmarried mothers served as a crystallisation point for these fears. From 1900 onwards a political impasse arose about the restructuring of filiation rules connected to paternity. Conservative evolutionary theory supplied the dogmatic solution for this impasse by stressing the universality and the 'naturalness' of marriage as an institution that creates fatherhood. The possibility that the granting of rights to mothers and duties to fathers outside marriage would undermine this condition, was averted by constructing a solution for the financial problems of illegitimate children outside family law, in the sphere of contract law. By a minor legal change in 1908, the begetter got the status of a debtor towards the child. The name of fatherhood was not attached to this status, because fatherhood was seen as a construction of family law. Lawyers, child protection agencies and charitable institutions for unmarried mothers became 'mediators' between illegitimate children, their mothers and the begetters. Unmarried mothers were denied automatic parental rights and rights to social services such as child allowances and pregnancy benefits, out of a fear that this would contaminate womanhood: the argument that the state should not encourage extra-matrimonial reproduction and licentiousness remained dominant until far into the twentieth century.

Thus, the unmarried mother was admitted to the legal order solely as a passive object, a target for the interference of the tutelary complex (Donzelot, 1979). In this way the patriarchal family, characterised by functional differentiation, hierarchy and 'unity' of the spouses, could remain the foundation of family law and the political order. The patriarchal institution of fatherhood was thus, for the time being, saved as the main point of reference in law, politics and citizenship. This coexisted with active and passive suffrage for all women from 1919. Public citizenship was thus introduced for women long before they became citizens in private law. Only in 1956 was the right to earnings and property for married women introduced in Holland, while the preferential legal position of fathers within marriage lasted until 1984.

NOTES

1 For that book I studied published documents that were linked to the campaigns about unmarried motherhood: political and legal journals, pamphlets, legal dissertations, sociological texts, law reform proposals, parliamentary debates and novels.

2 In my research I traced the emergence of the critique of the dual standard in several discourses. In feminist historiography the concept of the dual standard is often uncritically adapted as a explanatory and descriptive concept for feminist attitudes concerning sexuality, morality, and family law. In this way the contestations about the meanings of law and morality in the nineteenth century are hard to understand. To avoid these methodological problems I propose to see the concept of the dual standard as a critical strategic device, and to study the meaning it had for discussants in the debates on family law.

Chapter 9

Humanity or justice?
Wifebeating and the law in the eighteenth
and nineteenth centuries

Anna Clark

Public concern about wifebeating does not ebb and flow with the
actual incidence of the crime, but surges when domestic violence
becomes symbolically linked with other concerns (Gordon, 1989;
Pleck, 1987; Lambertz, 1990). Changes in the legal status of wifebeating therefore derive from changes in larger conceptions of
society and politics. In earlier eras, wifebeating was just one
example of the way in which superiors 'corrected' subordinates
through violence; but by the mid-nineteenth century, when
Parliament passed the first statute against wifebeating, violence in
general had become less acceptable and the state claimed a larger
role in regulating it.

Yet the law always treated wifebeating differently from other
assaults, hesitating to interfere in the private relations of man and
wife. The limited legal sanctions against domestic violence
functioned more to bolster the legitimacy of state power and
conventional marriage than to stop the crime. As marital ideals
shifted from classic seventeenth-century patriarchy to the softer
regime of nineteenth-century domesticity, the persistence of
wifebeating threatened the notion that men protected women in
the home. Furthermore, politicians blamed working-class disorder
for wifebeating, deflecting attention from the inequalities of
marriage itself.

At the same time, when put into practice, legal arenas became
'contested sites of power' which women tried to use for their own
ends (Smart, 1989: 138). Community morality and the battered
women's attempts to gain protection also shaped the everyday
practice of judges and magistrates (Ignatieff, 1983: 168). Communities sometimes interfered in egregious wifebeating, but
battered women usually had to rely on their own efforts to save

themselves. Economic circumstances could enable women to challenge their lack of legal rights, or constrain women to accept them. This article builds on much excellent previous work on the historical and contemporary causes of domestic violence, but concentrates on the interaction between legal changes and women's efforts to gain protection in the courts (Tomes, 1978; Ross, 1983; Lambertz, 1984; Gordon 1989; Dobash and Dobash, 1980; Pahl, 1985). Rather than take on the impossible task of quantifying the incidence of domestic violence, I will draw upon battered women's testimony in the courts as a qualitative source which reveals how such women positioned themselves in relation to the changing law.

Attitudes toward violence began to change from the seventeenth to the eighteenth centuries, a time of transition from a society justified by hierarchy and status to one justified by the social contract. According to the older conception of hierarchy, subjects obeyed the King, servants their masters, children their fathers and wives their husbands. Superiors could use violence as a tool to uphold hierarchy, as when the state executed criminals or parents corrected a child. Similarly, seventeenth-century society permitted husbands a certain latitude in 'correcting' their wives through force (Sharpe, 1983: 120). However, if a subordinate assaulted a superior, the courts would punish her for violating the social order. For instance, until 1790 wives who killed their husbands were burned at the stake for petty treason (Andrews [1881] 1980: 197).

Yet patriarchy, in the sense of men's domination of their wives and children, had its limits. Extreme, uncontrolled brutality would undermine patriarchy's legitimacy (Herrup, 1990: 12). As Susan Amussen points out, neighbours sometimes rescued battered wives or at least scolded violent husbands before the courts would ever intervene, but they may have waited to step in until the violence reached dangerous levels. Theologians advised husbands to dominate their wives through love and will rather than violence (Amussen, 1990: 5), but the courts very rarely punished wife-beating for most authorities held husbands had a right to correct their wives. Seventeenth-century judges only upheld the murder conviction of a man who beat his wife to death with a pestle because a pestle was a deadly weapon, not an appropriate instrument of correction (Russell, 1819, 1: 632, citing Crompton and Hale).

The realities of the family economy among middling and poor people also imposed limits, or at least strains, on patriarchy. Middling and working people often regarded marriage as a partnership, in which husband and wife shared the burdens of the productive family economy. Yet the economic importance of women clashed with a strongly patriarchal ideology (Underdown, 1985). Popular literature portrayed husbands and wives as 'struggling for the breeches', the prized trousers symbolising marital dominance (Clark, 1987: 228). Although women were supposed to submit, such literature suggested that men found it difficult to keep them from defying patriarchal authority. In response, communities subjected women who beat or otherwise dominated their husbands to the informal popular justice of rough music, publicly humiliating them by processing in front of their houses at night banging pots and pans (Thompson, 1972: 972; Malcolm, 1810: 205). One folklore authority pointed out that although this ritual was intended to humiliate women, some wives took it as a celebration of their belligerence (Brand, 1905, 2: 53).

Such marital struggles seemed plebeian to eighteenth-century legal authorities such as Blackstone, who observed in 1760 that since the reign of Charles II an increasingly polite society began to limit the legal extent of violence committed by a husband on his wife (Blackstone, 1793, 1: 444). Violence in general diminished and became less acceptable in the eighteenth century as sensibility and benevolence influenced English society (Beattie, 1986: 134).

Furthermore, Lockean social contract theory undermined the notion that society was based on natural subordination upheld by force, and attempted to replace it with the idea that free and equal individuals consented to the social order. In Locke's social compact, or contract as it is usually known, individuals consented to obey the law because it secured their rights and liberties (Harding, 1966: 296). This notion generated an ideology of equal justice under the law, as enshrined in the Bill of Rights, which in turn legitimated the social order after the Revolutionary Settlement of 1688. Of course, it remained a contentious notion, opposed by conservatives for its egalitarian connotations. Women and non-elite men could potentially apply the social contract's assumptions to themselves, as we shall see. Indeed, the challenge for the eighteenth-century legal system was how to retain the social contract's legitimising function without destroying the rank-and-gender hierarchies which structured British society. Blackstone, for instance, both celebrated the Bill of Rights' guarantee of the natural rights of Englishmen and remained attached to the principles of social hierarchy (Green, 1979: v).

In practice, only certain rights of certain people were protected. For instance, the courts and Parliament were much more interested in the rights of property than in protecting individuals from violence. Parliament multiplied the number of capital punishments for property offences while failing to remedy the law's lenience toward crimes against the person. In fact, attempted murder remained a misdemeanor, punishable by only a year and a day in gaol, until 1803. While Parliament passed over two hundred statutes mandating the death sentence for property crimes, it enacted only two felony statutes involving crimes against the person from the Restoration onward, and those in response to specific incidents of violence which threatened the authority of the monarch or the state. These statutes were so narrowly defined according to circumstance and type of injury that violent assaults on women short of murder were difficult to punish severely.[1]

The continuing contrast between the indifference to crimes of interpersonal violence and harshness toward property crimes was partially due to the social contract's implicit division of the world into public and private. The public sphere involved the relationship between the citizens and the government, while the private sector concerned relationships between individuals in business, civil society and personal life. The social contract between a citizen and government was inescapable, and if he violated the social order by committing felonies such as murder or robbery, the penalty was death. Relationships between individuals could be seen as contracts which would be dissolved or broken; the state simply regulated them as a service. Assaults between individuals or within families were seen as private matters, misdemeanors which the state punished lightly to ensure public peace (Beattie, 1986: 75–6). Nevertheless, even the most minor assault was technically illegal and people constantly prosecuted each other for pushing and shoving. Freedom from assault, declared Blackstone was a basic 'natural right' consisting of 'the right of personal security [which] consists in a person's legal and uninterrupted enjoyment of his life, his limbs, his body, his health, and his reputation' (Blackstone, 1793, 1:128).

However, legal authorities could not decide if women enjoyed this right, if the social contract applied to them as well. Blackstone's sanctions on wifebeating simply meant that the law limited the degree of violence a husband could inflict, rather than prohibiting wifebeating altogether. Whipping and cudgelling were no longer acceptable means of correction, but Hawkins and other legal authorities said a husband could beat his wife 'though not outrageously' (cited in Kenny, 1879: 153). Furthermore, Sir Francis Buller's alleged pronouncement in 1783 that a man could beat his wife with a stick no bigger than his thumb, although never a legal precedent, certainly entered popular belief.[2] In one case, Hale refuted the notion that a husband could violently correct his wife, but in 1736 Bacon wrote that a husband could enforce his wife's duty by beating her 'but not in a violent or cruel manner' (Doggett, 1990: 4).

These authorities were so vague because of the contradictions of social contract theory when applied to women. In fact, Locke began his genesis of the 'social compact' by contrasting it with the original compact between men and women. In his eagerness to undermine ideas of natural subordination, he limited a husband's powers by conceiving of marriage as a contract. However, he also wished to differentiate between relations within the family – where he still regarded (albeit limited) subordination as based on nature – from political relations between men, which were based on free consent between equals (Locke, 1967, 2: 339, 350). As Susan Staves argues, property lawyers at first applied contract theory by regarding women as free individuals in marriage contracts, but later in the eighteenth century, judges began to reverse this trend, because it undermined women's subordination within marriage (Staves, 1990: 229).

Carole Pateman explains this paradox by considering marriage as a sexual contract which parallels the social contract (Pateman, 1989). In the sexual contract, women consented to obey their husbands in return for protection. Women supposedly did not need individual rights because their husbands protected them; as Pateman points out, they consented to surrender their rights in an inescapable contract, unlike any other contract between citizens. The division between public and private was further refined by the developing ideology of separate spheres, in which men belonged to the dominant public sphere of work and politics, and women sheltered, safe and submissive, in the domestic private sphere of the home (Davidoff and Hall, 1987). And given that the domestic private sphere was seen as separate from the state, the role of the state in regulating it was ambiguous (Engelstein, 1988: 458). On the one hand, since the state had the duty only to redress public wrongs, i.e. injuries which threatened the social order, wifebeating was not a matter of state concern because it occurred in the private world of the home. On the other hand, the point of the social contract was to abjure the idea of 'might makes right'. The emphasis on consent represented a change from the old rank-and-gender hierarchy, where violence could be used to enforce submission. The marriage contract was also based on consent – but as Pateman points out, consent to subordination.

Such ambiguities explain the confusion of legal authorities such as Hawkins and Blackstone, who theoretically limited a husband's right to beat his wife, but hesitated to allow women effective redress against brutal spouses. Wives could swear out an article of the peace (similar to an injunction) against abusive husbands, but obtaining these documents required 'considerable charge and trouble', in Defoe's words, and often failed in their purpose (Pahl, 1985: 95). Burns vaguely advised magistrates that 'some say' a man could 'correct' or 'chastise' his wife without forfeiting his sureties under an article of the peace (Burns, 1776, 4: 268). However, it was unclear if women actually had the right to prosecute their husbands and testify against them as witnesses, because of the general principle that spouses could not testify against each other. In 1764, the Middlesex justices admitted 'they were greatly at a loss' on this matter, but eventually decided against wives.[3]

However, the justices had to decide on this matter because they faced continual pressure from wives who wished to prosecute their husbands for assault whether or not they had a right to do so. In fact, since at least the early eighteenth century, women brought their husbands before magistrates and charged them with assault.[4] By the 1780s and 90s, at least one woman a week appeared before the Middlesex Justices to prosecute her husband (or common-law spouse) for assault. And in the 1790s, the magistrates occasionally found some of these husbands guilty on the sole evidence of their wives.[5]

How were these battered wives able to find the courage to go to the court in the face of legal indifference? The answer lies in the fact that late-eighteenth-century plebeian London women did not live according to the conventional notions of the sexual contract. Since they helped in family businesses or sometimes ran their own shops, or worked at needlework, laundry or other trades, many did not passively depend on their husbands' protection. Working and socialising in London streets, they blurred the divisions between public and private dictated by the middle-class conventions of separate spheres (Clark, 1987: 24). Their experience in public life apparently gave them greater confidence to appear in court than their rural sisters enjoyed. Like male Londoners, they were notoriously litigious, eagerly prosecuting for assault when insulted or assaulted (Landau, 1984: 197). Although they did not have full rights as propertied citizens, they enthusiastically believed in equal justice under the laws (Thompson, 1975: 264).

Despite the ambivalence of legal authorities toward battered wives, some of the women who testified in court or submitted articles of the peace espoused faith that the law would protect them. When a militia sergeant asked his estranged wife to withdraw the article of the peace she had served against him, she told him:

> that the regard she owed both herself and him would make her take the security of the law against him for ill-usage from him in the future, being convinced, that if she did not, he would at last be the death of her.
>
> (*Universal Register (Times)* 15 October 1788)

Susannah Hunt wrote in her article of the peace that her former common-law husband, a gentleman, had threatened to murder her so many times that she feared he will 'carry his threats into Execution if he discovers where this Exhibitant is unless restrained by the authority of the law'.[6]

However, plebeian women still faced the tension between their own understanding of the marital contract and the law which constrained them. The experience of carrying on a craft or trade on their own or with their husbands may have led to a view of marriage as a businesslike partnership rather than a contract of submission and dependence (Gillis, 1985: 175). If their husbands battered them, wives in such situations could envision their lost independence and hope to regain it. But no matter how hardworking and confident, wives had no legal control over their own wages and property. Some women went to court because they resented their loss of property and independence as well as their husbands' violence.[7] For instance, Catherine Rolph complained that her husband, a shopkeeper, not only beat her but forced her to give him the money she had earned selling stock-neckties.[8] Elizabeth Sims asked a magistrate for a separation because 'in the absence of her husband, which frequently happened for a some considerable time, she did very well, and got forward, but whenever he returned, he beat her, spent her money, and threatened her life' (*The Times* 21 April 1801). Similarly, Ann Casson deposed 'prior to her intermarriage . . . she kept a grocers' shop in Edgeware Road and was doing very well when she unfortunately became acquainted with and met her said husband who had little or no property at all.'[9] For such women, husbands represented more of a liability than an asset. Yet many plebeian battered women who worked for their husbands or depended on them found themselves trapped in a very different situation. These women feared that if their husbands left as a result of a prosecution (or in very rare cases, were imprisoned for short terms), they would lose most of their economic support.

Perhaps as a result, plebeian women seem to have hesitated to charge abusive husbands. Evidence for this lies in the fact that the number of cases in which women prosecuted unrelated men for minor assaults far outnumbered cases of wifebeating, though it is likely that the amount of wifebeating was actually much greater. Women prosecuted other men for offences such as hair-pulling, 'pulling about', threats, and water-throwing, which implies that they believed they could use the law to protect against any assault. But women who prosecuted husbands, and the clerks who drew up articles of the peace and indictments, justified their cases by emphasising that beatings were exceptionally severe, or 'inhuman'. An indictment against a St Giles labourer for assault against his wife, Johanna Donnovan, accused him of 'ill-treat[ing] her in an outrageous and inhuman manner'.[10] Similarly, the indictment against John Gaskin, a winecooper, for threatening to murder his wife with a sword stated he had committed an 'inhuman' assault on her.[11] At the Guildhall magistrates court, Mary Taylor accused her husband of 'treating her with so much inhumanity' by 'keeping company with naughty women . . . and depriving her of the necessities of life' (*Universal Register (Times)* 10 January 1785).

According to her sister, a Mr Emberson beat his wife 'inhumanly', leading Mary Emberson to seek a divorce.[12]

In the eighteenth century, the word 'humanity' derived from Christian charity, but it also meant being humane, as in polite and well-mannered, and sympathetically recognising the common humanity of others (*Oxford English Dictionary*; Williams, 1983: 149). Judges told men convicted of the murder or manslaughter of their wives that they were 'unmanly' or 'inhuman'; it was 'an attack made by the strong on the weak', for 'instead of using her cruelly himself, he ought to be her Protector from ill-treatment by others'.[13] By regarding wifebeating as a violation of chivalrous politesse, rather than as violation of women's rights, legal authorities further excluded women from the social contract. As Hume stated, women had no absolute claim to the rules of justice, since they were 'too weak to resist wrong', but 'humanity' and manners enabled them to share in rights and privileges in civilised society (Hume, 1965: 42). Women appealed to the protectionism of the sexual contract, but the sexual contract only gave them protection on suffrance, not as individuals with rights. Only 'inhuman' brutality would be punished, not everyday punches and slaps.

Magistrates also cited 'humanity' to justify their efforts to mediate assault cases, believing reconciliation could prevent further violence through mediation (Hawkins, 1780: 2). As anthropologists have noted, mediation generally functions to restore hierarchy within communities, rather than to uphold equality (Abel, 1982: 4; Castan, 1983: 255). This was especially true in cases of wifebeating, for magistrates had to persuade wives who had been beaten to return to their assailants, therefore buttressing the patriarchal order of marriage. Furthermore, contemporary studies of wifebeating have found that mediation is ineffectual in preventing further assaults (Pahl, 85: 185).

Even if they did not desire mediation, people went to court to air their grievances, as anthropologists have found (Roberts, 1983: 23). No doubt some women went to court to shame their husbands and to denounce wifebeating in a public arena, often with the support of other women. And communities in the late-eighteenth century began to shame violent husbands as well as termagant wives, according to E.P. Thompson (1972: 980). However, rough music was a rare event, while wifebeating occurred everyday, and the many men who believed they had the right to beat their wives could not be so shamed. For instance, Mordecai Moses, charged together with his mistress for beating his wife, would 'make no promise of good behaviour' and 'only offered a series of recriminations in his defence'.[14] Magistrates could reprimand violent husbands and order them to apologise, but after such public humiliation they were unlikely to treat their wives well back at home. For instance, when Ann Casson charged her husband with assault, the magistrate 'talked a great deal to him, and as he then seemed very sorry for what he had done, and as he promised to behave better in the future they advised a reconciliation which took place immediately'. Soon after, Casson 'used her worse than before, and threatened to dash her brains out with a poker'.[15] Women such as Ann Casson struggled to use the law for their own ends, but their husbands defied the half-hearted attempts of the law to restrain them and seized the privileges of the sexual contract instead.

By the beginning of the nineteenth century, however, the weakness of the laws against assaults in general began to threaten the legitimacy of the state as violent offenders escaped with light sentences. Inspired by the French Revolution, radicals declared that the discrepancy between harsh penalties for property crimes and leniency towards violence proved that the law excluded all but the propertied from its benefits (Linebaugh, 1975: 65). In response to these threats to state authority, Parliament passed Lord Ellenborough's Acts in 1803, which imposed death sentences for the first time on attempted murder and grievous bodily harm.

But the old system of terror could not suppress political turbulence and violence in general. Instead, the state moved toward more extensive regulation of violence as the middle class, motivated by evangelicalism and humanitarianism, demanded rational, efficient protection. Middle-class men rejected the old notion of honour and hierarchy defended by violence; instead, they espoused rationality and self-control, achieving manhood through hard work in the public sphere rather than aggression within personal relations (Davidoff and Hall, 1987: 21). Furthermore, for the middle class, private morality necessarily accompanied public, political virtue. While they upheld the sanctity of their own homes, they believed that they should interfere in the private lives of working people, for the perceived disorder and crime in working-class families and communities threatened society as a whole. Violence thus acquired a symbolic currency in political discourse, for middle-class men pointed to their own self-control as a justification for their claims to political power, while attacking the working class as too violent to deserve the vote. In response to these concerns, by the 1830s, police surveillance and long prison sentences replaced the threat of death as the means for the state to regulate violence (Radzinowicz, 1948, 1: 583). By 1837, the death penalty was removed from grievous bodily harm in order to increase the prosecution and conviction rates for this offence.

The new protectionist intrusion into working-class lives had ambiguous consequences for women. The law now offered women potential protection from violence through the police and through greater sanctions against serious assaults. But it also diminished women's control over the prosecution process. And women's increasing economic dependency limited their ability to envision prison for their husbands. By the mid-nineteenth century, working-class wives were less likely to work outside of the home, and female occupations were scarce and miserably paid (Alexander, 1976). Despite these constraints, some battered wives still struggled to use the law for their own ends. They found that different levels of the criminal justice system varied in their responsiveness to women: from the police, to the magistrates courts, which settled cases or passed them on to the higher courts; finally to the Old Bailey, the London higher court where juries tried felony cases.

Battered women could now call upon the police for help during an assault, but the police, then as now, probably refused to interfere in most cases of domestic violence. In 1834, the radical *Weekly Dispatch* complained of the 'Inefficiency of the New Police' who were nowhere to be seen when a husband chased his wife into the street and beat her with a poker (21 December 1834). Women also faced the continuing ambivalence towards the police within the community. In 1830, the *Weekly Dispatch* indignantly exposed the 'Over Officiousness of the New Police' who charged a man with 'quarrelling with his own wife!' (12 December 1830) Regarding the police as outsiders, some women resented their attempts to interfere.

However, women could go directly to the magistrates courts for a warrant and bypass the police constables. Nineteenth-century Londoners in general and battered women in particular seem to have resorted to the magistrates courts with enthusiasm. For instance, Elizabeth Cooney demanded protection one week after marriage because her husband 'tyrannised' over her (*Weekly Dispatch* 25 July 1841). As Jennifer Davis writes, working-class people expected the magistrates courts to provide them with justice on their own terms and regarded the legal system as oppressive when they did not (Davis, 1984: 310). In fact, the jurisdiction of the magistrates courts over assaults was extended in 1828, due to popular demand, especially from 'disputes between man and wife' (Commissioners on Police 1828: 147). Although magistrates could now impose 2-month gaol sentences for assault, they continued to focus on mediation rather than punishment. In 1837 magistrate Rawlinson told Martha Taylor to reconcile with her husband, a journeyman paper hanger, after he beat her. She declared in a passion, 'Make it up! Never! I'll suffer death first!'. When asked what she wished the magistrate to do, she asked the magistrate to bind him up 'neck and heels to keep the peace, or let him go to prison if he can't find bail'. The magistrate, however, only bound him over to keep the peace on his own recognisance, asserting there were 'faults on both sides' (*London Mercury* 22 January 1837). As this example reveals, the magistrates varied in their willingness to provide protection. Furthermore, even if the full sentence were imposed, 2 months was not long for very serious assaults.

Although women could prosecute husbands who committed grievous bodily harm in the Old Bailey Sessions, where judges could impose sentences of several years' duration, they seemed reluctant to do so. Old Bailey judges were concerned with demonstrating state control over violence and crime, and they intimidated battered women. Even if women initially wished to prosecute, the great expense and trouble, the likelihood that their husbands would promise reform in the intervening time and their economic dependency often produced an ambivalence which comes through in the Old Bailey testimony of battered wives. The police could also now prosecute violent husbands even if their victims were unwilling, so that women who earlier would not have sought protection were now forced to testify in the well-documented Old Bailey Sessions. For instance, when William New was tried for stabbing his wife Sarah, she testified 'I do not think he meant to hurt me', and refused even to appear before the magistrate. It was the police who arrested him and committed him for trial. Her ambivalence may have had something to do with the fact that she was out of work at the time, and therefore needed his support.[16] Bridget Barrett, whose husband kicked her while she was pregnant, testified, 'I know he did not intend to injure me – I wish to grant his pardon as much as possible – I have a child 5 years old, and we are dependent on him.'[17]

Women's interests in gaining separations and the court's interests in imposing punishment conflicted. Ellen Donovan declared, 'I do not wish to hurt him – I only want peace and quiet and a maintenance.' But her testimony also reveals a typical conflict between self-blame and desire for revenge. At first she said that his beating, which put her in the hospital for 2 weeks, was 'perhaps ... my fault as much as his,' but after he insulted her in the trial, she burst out, 'he is a great murderer, and I should like him punished ... and I should not have given him in charge now but for the women in the same house.'[18] Alone, she could not have stood up for herself, but the other women did not want to see a violent husband go free (Ross, 1983: 580; Tomes, 1978: 332).

By the 1840s, the reluctance of wives to prosecute and juries to convict for domestic violence threatened to undermine the legitimacy of the law, complained law-and-order advocates in a public newspaper debate (May, 1978: 143). *The Times* noted indignantly that a man who beat and tried to strangle his wife was convicted only of common assault, though he had previously threatened to kill her (24 August 1846). The *Daily News* pointed out 'how much safer it is to stab one's wife than to defraud one's master'(24 August 1846). However, the solution for this injustice, according to the journalists, was to remove domestic violence from the conventions of the common law of manslaughter and murder and increase chivalrous state control over prosecutions. Some commentators felt frustrated at the reluctance of women to prosecute violent husbands, and wished to take this decision out of women's hands. 'A Lover of Justice' wrote that:

It is worth serious consideration on the part of legislators to see whether a law may not be framed to meet these cases – to remove from the tender hands of the wife the power of shielding a ruffianly husband from the offended laws.

(*Reynolds Newspaper* 21 December 1851)

The *Daily News* argued that wifekilling should be defined as manslaughter because juries refused to return verdicts of murder despite clear evidence of express malice; if the crime were defined as manslaughter, argued the paper, at least there would be a greater chance of a conviction (28 August 1846, also *The Times* 22 July 1847). Manslaughter was homicide caused by provocation, and did not incur the death penalty. By defining all wifekillings as manslaughter, this proposal implicitly judged wifekilling not as a violation of an individual's rights under the the social contract, but by the different standards of the sexual contract. A man's duty was to protect, and a wife's to submit. If he killed her, it could be excused as provocation, and the full public sanction would not fall on him.

In 1853 Parliament contended with the tension between the desire to protect women and the principles of the law by passing a measure against wifebeating while rejecting reform and codification of the wider criminal law. The reluctance of women to prosecute and juries to convict in higher courts, and the inadequacy of the sentences magistrates could impose, impelled legislators to adopt the Aggravated Assaults on Women and Children Act, which allowed magistrates to impose 6 months' sentences for such crimes. But Parliament opposed the Criminal Law Commissioners' recommendations to replace the irrationalities and discrepancies of the wider law on crimes of violence against persons with a rational code exactly proportioning prison sentences to the severity of crimes. Legislators believed such increased state regulation of violence could infringe upon the rights of English men. They asserted it deprived both victims and judges of their discretion in assessing the severity of assault, and moreover, smacked of French despotism and imperialism in India (Manchester, 1973: 410; Hostettler, 1984: 2). But Parliament showed no such resistance to extending the power of magistrates to impose relatively long sentences upon wifebeaters convicted without jury trials.

The creation of a 'moral panic' around wifebeating was another reason why the Aggravated Assault Act succeeded while codification failed. Codification required sustained, unglamorous political effort, while Parliament preferred to react to 'moral panics' about crime, such as garotting or obscenity (Davis, 1980: 205; Roberts, 1985: 630). Moral concerns about wifebeating became symbolically linked to political debates over the citizenship of women and working-class men. Parliament overcame its long opposition to interfering in the private sphere of the home by defining wifebatterers as working-class brutes who did not deserve the right to privacy and their victims as passive creatures who could not determine their own fates. During working-class agitation, conservatives often attacked the morality of the working class in order to discredit their claims to suffrage. If working men were irresponsible husbands, they could not claim the privilege of the vote. The conservative religious journal *The British Workman*, dedicated to turning working men away from radical action, told them: 'Gentlemen, there are two ways of governing a family: the first is by force, the other is by mild and vigilant authority .... A husband deserves to lose his empire altogether, by making an attempt to force it with violence' (1 October 1855). Working men therefore had to earn the privilege of control over women, just as the journal admonished them to prove their respectability before they demanded political rights.

As Jan Lambertz has written, the middle-class press insisted on seeing wifebeating as symptomatic of working-class degradation, which could only be alleviated through top-down measures such as severe punishments, or, conversely, education (Lambertz, 1984: 79). In an editorial on wifebeating *The Times* fulminated against the lower classes as 'a race of barbarians, ignorant alike of their duty to God and man, and stimulating the most ferocious passions by the most brutal excesses'. It called for education to 'elevate' the lower orders, but went on to say that 'if we will not teach we must punish, and the lessons which ought to be impressed by reason must be inculcated by fear' in the form of flogging of wifebeaters (20 August 1852). The wifebeater was now a brutal other of the urban lower depths, who could only be treated with terror, not rational regulation.

Furthermore, by attributing wifebeating solely to working-class brutes, newspaper and Parliamentary debate displaced the problem of male violence on to class. In an era when feminism was just beginning to be heard, the intense publicity over wifebeating potentially undermined the legitimacy of the patriarchal sexual contract, in which men's dominance was justified by their protection of their wives. Attempting to justify women's legal disabilities in marriage, J.J.S. Wharton explained: 'Private government in conjugal society, arrives at ... perfection, where ... the man bears rule over his wife's person and conduct, she bears rule over his inclinations, he governs by law, she by persuasion' (Wharton, 1853: 467, quoting Lord Kaimes). If persuasion failed, women had no status in law. The polemicist Caroline Norton had long ago pointed out this paradox, arguing that when a man beat his wife, 'he is no longer the administrator and exponent of the law, but its direct opponent' (Norton, 1978: 167). Another middle-class writer on women's issues, Caroline Napier, declared that a false notion of male authority:

> leads men to indulge their tempers at the expense of female happiness, who would shrink from doing so, if they saw their conduct in the light of injustice, or discerned that their claim to submission rested on no better basis than force.
>
> (Napier, 1844: 201)

She asserted that women had the right to protection from abuse on the basis of justice, not merely humanity. But both Norton and Napier persisted in upholding the principle that the male is the head of the household and rightfully dominant. Thus, wifebeating could be criticised without challenging patriarchy itself.

In contrast, as Lambertz states, feminists such as Harriet Taylor Mill and John Stuart Mill asserted that women lacked adequate protection from the law because they were deprived of their rights as citizens in the social contract (Lambertz, 1984: 80). An editorial in the *Morning Chronicle* by Taylor and Mill explained women's reluctance to prosecute by declaring that punishments are so inadequate women feel it is useless to pursue a case. The editorial pointed out that 'At present it is very well known that women, in the lower ranks of life, do not expect justice from a bench or jury of the male sex' (28 October 1846). Mill and Taylor also critiqued marriage itself, for as another editorial proclaimed, 'The vow to protect thus confers a licence to kill' (*Morning Chronicle* 28 August 1851). And Harriet Taylor Mill went beyond the sexual contract of marriage, declaring that women would only be safe if they did not depend economically on their husbands (Mill, 1970: 105).

Of course, the Aggravated Assaults on Women and Children Act did not change the rules of marriage, and it only punished those men who violated the sexual contract by using force, rather moral authority, to rule. It had a limited effect because wives could not fully prosecute their husbands if they were financially dependent on them. When they appeared before the magistrates courts, sometimes mangled and bloody, they still testified reluctantly. Women apologised for their husbands' beatings by saying 'he was in liquor', or 'he was not in the habit of ill-using her'. One woman began with these excuses, explaining her injury by saying her husband's foot 'slipped' on her stomach, but later admitted he had kicked her and often beat her. The magistrates' action in committing him for 6 months would protect her from assault, but also deprive her of a breadwinner (*The Times* 5 January 1854). Furthermore, magistrates tended to judge wives according to the rule of the sexual contract; although this pattern varied by the individual justice, they would extend protection to a passive, meek wife who conformed to her obligation to obey, while stigmatising the assertive wife as shrewish and deserving of punishment (Lambertz, 1984: 81–5; Tomes, 1978: 344; Ross, 1983: 591). As a result, the Act was mainly used to punish violence committed by men on women and children unrelated to them (Returns Relating to Assaults on Women and Children, 1854–1855).

The limited efficacy of the Act led to further calls for reform, but feminists and law-and-order advocates proposed contrasting solutions. In 1856, a Parliamentary measure allowing flogging of wifebeaters stirred up public indignation at 'unmanly brutes', but the women of Leicester opposed it, fearing it would inspire men to even worse violence and therefore deter women from prosecuting (Kaye, 1856: 256). Feminists argued that separation and maintenance orders would be more useful in allowing women to escape violent men without losing their source of subsistence. Although an Act enabling this was eventually passed in 1878, magistrates often refused separation orders, and the problem of wifebeating continued (Lambertz, 1984: 81). While Nancy Tomes cites statistics to show that the crime declined considerably during the late-nineteenth century, even as the means for prosecuting husbands expanded, Ellen Ross argues that wifebeating continued to be very common in the late-nineteenth century (Tomes, 1978: 345; Ross, 1983: 590).

CONCLUSION

Changing laws concerning wifebeating symbolise and legitimate the changing nature of patriarchal control over women in the family, and of the state's control over its citizens. In the seventeenth century, violence by husbands paralleled state violence as legitimate means of correcting subordinates. Popular culture, however, reveals that women were difficult to keep down. In the eighteenth century, the sexual contract paralleled the social contract, promising citizens and women protection in exchange for obedience. In practice, the law rarely protected women and allowed private patriarchy to continue, but the gap between ideal and reality was apparent to the women who took their husbands to court. In the nineteenth century, state interference in wifebeating ensured the legitimacy of the law and a new form of domestic patriarchy in which control over women was to be rational, not physical. Legislators attempted to criticise wifebeaters as working-class brutes to deflect feminist challenges to patriarchal marriage and indeed women and working men's claims to citizenship. Today, wifebeating is a public concern, but increasingly defined as gender-neutral 'domestic violence' rather than as a matter of patriarchal power.

Yet battered wives themselves could attempt to use these changing laws in order to gain protection. It is important – for the historical record and for the present – to remember and hear what women want and how they articulate their needs, not just how the law oppresses them. Accounts of eighteenth- and nineteenth-century battered wives evoke many of the dilemmas we face today: how to empower women by asking what they want from the courts, while facing the fact that many women drop charges and blame themselves. They also illuminate, but complicate, current debates on the ability of dominant discourses to structure totally women's ability to articulate their grievances and gain protection from the courts and social services (Gordon, 1990; Scott, 1990). The experience of economic independence clearly enabled some women to challenge eighteenth-century patriarchal norms and demand protection from abusive husbands. But other women adopted the dominant discourses, whether as a strategy – portraying assaults as exceptionally 'inhuman' in order to gain judges' sympathy – or as internalised oppression – when wives blamed themselves for assaults against them. We must admire the courage of the women who could defy patriarchy, while recognising the power of the law to frustrate their efforts. Even today, economic independence helps women be assertive in the courts, but it does not guarantee their protection from male violence.

ACKNOWLEDGEMENTS

I wish to thank the American Bar Foundation, the Law and Social Science Program of Northwestern University and the Foundation of the University of North Carolina at Charlotte for funding the research for this essay. I would also like to thank Judith Walkowitz and Olwen Hufton for comments on the very earliest germs of this paper, Jan Lambertz for generously sharing her important unpublished thesis, Maeve Doggett and Susan Amussen for sending me unpublished papers, and Julia Blackwelder, Amy Thomas, Cynthia Herrup, and Carol Smart for their astute comments on its current incarnation.

NOTES

1 According to Adam Smith, during a House of Commons debate on a playhouse, some members alleged it was kept for the King's amusement. Sir John Coventry asked whether this was meant of the male or female players. This enraged the court party, and at the King's desire the Duke of Monmouth and some others waylaid Sir John and slit his nose and ears. In response the House of Commons passed the Coventry Acts, which made it a felony to lie in wait and maim or disfigure (Smith, 1978: 118). However, when a man who slit his wife's throat as she lay sleeping was indicted under the Coventry Acts at the Old Bailey Sessions in 1763, his assault was held not to fall under the act as he did not 'lay in wait' or disfigure or maim her (Leach's Crown Cases, vol. I, p. 52. Lee's case). The only other statutes involving violence were the Black Acts of 1723 making shooting a felony, in response to woodlands disturbances and possible Jacobitism (Thompson, 1975). But in the eighteenth century firearms were very rarely used in domestic violence.

2 Simpson (1984: 88) says Buller did not originate the phrase, but it reflected his personal attitude; Townsend (1846) states that Buller 'unpremeditatedly' blurted out the phrase. For popular views, see *Ramblers' Magazine* (London, 1783), I: 35. Officially overturned in R.v. Jackson (Pahl, 1985: 11).

3 Greater London Record Office (GLRO) Middlesex Justices Order Book, MJ/OC/8 18 October 1764: 3.

4 GLRO, Henry Norris's Daybook, 1730–1748, M79/x/1.

5 Cases: GLRO, Middlesex Sessions, 1791, Tillerson, Roll 3529, Indictment 4; Moody, Roll 3538, Indictment 54; 1792, Pageter, Roll 3550, Indictment 54; Harris, Roll 3553, Indictment 28.

6 GLRO 1792, Hunt, Roll 3545, Indictment 48.

7 Margaret Hunt similarly found that middle-class women with financial and familial resources were the ones who tried to divorce their husbands (Hunt, 1988: 2).

8 GLRO, Middlesex Sessions, 1781, Roll 3406, unnumbered article of the peace.

9 GLRO, Middlesex Sessions 1795, Roll 3582, Indictment 32; for similar testimony, Ann Barras's article of the peace, 1793, Roll 3563, Indictment 57; Martha Seldon's article of the peace, 1792, Roll 3553, Indictment 47.

10 GLRO Middlesex Sessions, 1792, Roll 3548, Indictment 71.

11 GLRO, Middlesex Sessions 1792, Roll 3548, Indictment 43.

12 GLRO, London Consistory Court, DL/C 281, 27 November 1780, Emberson v. Emberson.

13 Old Bailey Sessions Papers, October 1790, 944 and December 1790, 2; trial of Albert Lowe, 1780, in Alsatian Eccentricities, a collection of clippings in the British Library.

14 Unusually, and perhaps due to the immorality of his keeping a mistress, the magistrate committed him for want of sureties (bail). City of London Record Office, Guildhall Justice Room Minute Books, 17 September 1783; similar case 7 February 1796.

15 GLRO, Middlesex Sessions 1795, Roll 3582, Indictment 32.

16 Old Bailey Session Papers, 20 September 1844, 3: 771.

17 Old Bailey Sessions Papers, 1 December 1842, 1 (1842–3): 16–18.

18 Old Bailey Sessions Papers, 6 April 1843, 2: 994.

References

Abbot, P. and Wallace, C. (1989) 'The family', in P. Brown and R. Sparks (eds) *Beyond Thatcherism*, London: Open University Press, p. 78.

Abel, R. (1982) Introduction, *The Politics of Informal Justice*, R. Abel (ed.) Vol. 1, *The American Experience*, New York: Academic Press.

Abelson, E.S. (1989) *When Ladies Go A-Thieving*, Oxford: Oxford University Press.

Alexander, S. (1976) 'Women's work in nineteenth century London: a study of the years 1820–1850', in J. Mitchell and A. Oakley (eds) *The Rights and Wrongs of Women*, Harmondsworth: Penguin.

Allen, H. (1987) *Justice Unbalanced*, Milton Keynes: Open University Press.

Amussen, S.D. (1990) 'Violence and domestic violence in early modern England', paper presented at the Berkshire Conference of Women Historians.

Andrews, W. [1881] (1980) *Old-Time Punishments*, Toronto: Coles.

Antrobus, P. (1964) 'Coloured children in care – a special problem group?' *Case Conference* June, 11(2): 39–45.

Arnup, K. (1990) 'Educating mothers: government advice for women in the inter-war years', in K. Arnup, A. Levesque and R.R. Pierson (eds) *Delivering Motherhood: Maternal Ideologies and Practices in the 19th and 20th Centuries*, London: Routledge.

Bachofen, J.J. (1861) *Das Mutterrecht. Eine Untersuchung über die Gynaikokratie der Alten Welt nach ihrer religiosen und rechtlichen Natur*, Stuttgart.

Bailey, V. and Blackburn, S. (1979) 'The Punishment of Incest Act 1908: a case study of law creation', *Criminal Law Review* 708–18.

Bailey, V. and McCabe, S. (1979) 'Reforming the Law of Incest', *Criminal Law Review* 749–64.

Baker, P. (1984) 'The domestication of politics: women and American political society, 1780–1920', *American Historical Review* 89.

Banks, O. (1981) *Faces of Feminism*, Oxford: Martin Robertson.

Barnett, H. (1881) *The Work of Lady Visitors*, London: Metropolitan Association for Befriending Young Servants.

Beattie, J.M. (1986) *Crime and the Courts in England, 1660–1800*, Oxford: Oxford University Press.

Bebel, A. (1897) *Die Frau und der Sozialismus*, Stuttgart.

Behlmer, G.K. (1979) 'Deadly motherhood: infanticide and medical opinion in mid-Victorian England', *Journal of the History of Medicine* 34: 403–27.

Behlmer, G.K. (1982) *Child Abuse and Moral Reform in England 1870–1908*, Stanford: Stanford University Press.

Bentovim, A., Elton, A. and Tranter, M. (1987) 'Prognosis for rehabilitation after abuse', *Adoption & Fostering* 11(1): 26–31.

Berton, P. (1977) *The Dionne Years*, Toronto: McClelland & Stewart.

Best, G. (1964) *Temporal Pillars*, Cambridge: Cambridge University Press.

Beveridge, W. (1942) *Social Insurance and Allied Services*, London: HMSO, Cmd 6404.

Blackstone, W. (1793) *Commentaries on the Laws of England*, 12th ed., with notes by Edward Christian, 4 vols.

Blackwell, E. (1881) *Rescue in Work in Relation to Prostitution and Disease*, London.

Blackwell, E. (1887) *Purchase of Women: the Great Economic Blunder*, London: John Kensit.

Bland, L. (1982) '"Guardians of the race" or "vampires upon the nation's health?" Female sexuality and its regulation in early 20C Britain', in E. Whitelegg, M. Arnot, E. Bartels, V. Beechey, L. Birke, S. Himmelweit, D. Leonard, S. Ruehl and M.A. Speakman (eds) *The Changing Experience of Women*, Oxford: Basil Blackwell.

Bland, L. (1983) 'Purity, motherhood, pleasure or threat? Definitions of female sexuality 1900–1970s', in S. Cartledge and J. Ryan (eds) *Sex & Love*, London: The Women's Press.

Bland, L. (1985) 'In the name of protection: the policing of women in the First World War', in C. Smart and J. Brophy (eds) *Women in Law: Explorations in Law, Family and Sexuality* London: Routledge & Kegan Paul.

Blatz, W. (1938) *The Five Sisters: A Study in Child Psychology*, Toronto: University of Toronto Press.

Blatz, W. *et al.* (1937) *Collected Studies on the Dionne Quintuplets*, Toronto: University of Toronto Press.

Bosanquet, H. (1896) *Rich and Poor*, London: Macmillan.

Bosanquet, H. (1897) 'The Psychology of Social Progress', *International Journal of Ethics* VII (April).

Bosanquet, H. (1898a) *The Standard of Life and Other Studies*, London: Macmillan.

Bosanquet, H. (1898b) *The Administration of Charitable Relief*, London: National Union of Women Workers.

Bosanquet, H. (1900) 'Methods of Training', *Charity Organisation Review* (August) pp. 103–9.

Bosanquet, H. (1903) *The Strength of the People, A Study in Social Economics*, London: Macmillan.

Bosanquet, H. (1906) *The Family*, London: Macmillan.

Bowlby, J. (1940) 'Psychological aspects, evacuation survey: a report to the Fabian Society', in R. Padley and M. Cole (eds) *Evacuation Survey*, London: George Routledge & Sons.

Bowlby, J. (1953) *Child Care and the Growth of Love*, London: Pelican Books.

Brand, J. (1905) *Popular Antiquities*, London, 2 vols.

Braybon, G. and Summerfield, P. (1987) *Out of the Cage*, London: Pandora.

Brennan, T. and Pateman, C. (1979) 'Mere auxiliaries to the Common-wealth. Women and the origins of liberalism', *Political Studies* XXVII (2): 183–200.

Bristow, E. (1977) *Vice and Vigilance*, Dublin: Gill & Macmillan.

Brough, J. (1965) *We Were Five*, New York: Bantam.

Buchholz, S. (1979) 'Savigny's Stellungnahme zum Ehe-und Familien-recht', *Ius Commune* 8: 148–91.

Burdett Coutts (1893) *Women's Mission to Women*, London: Sampson Low Marston & Co.

Burlingham, D. and Freud, A. (1942) *Young Children in War-time: A Year's Work in a Residential War Nursery*, London: Allen & Unwin.

Burns, R. (1776) *Justice of the Peace*, London, 4 vols.

Burrow, J. (1970) *Evolution and Society. A Study in Victorian Social Theory*, Cambridge: Cambridge University Press.

Butler, J. (1897) quoted in Higson, J. (1955) *The Story of a Beginning*, London: SPCK.

Butler, J (1990) *Gender Trouble*, London: Routledge.

Carlen, P (1983) *Women's Imprisonment*, London: Routledge & Kegan Paul.

Castan, N. (1983) 'The arbitration of disputes under the old regime', in J. Bossy (ed.) *Disputes and Settlements*, Cambridge: Cambridge University Press.

Chant, L. (1888) *The Vigilance Record*, January.

Chant, L. (1889) *The Vigilance Record*, April.

Chant, L. (1894a) *The Women's Signal*, 1 November.

Chant, L. (1894b) *The Vigilance Record*, November.

Chant, L. (1895) *Why We Attacked the Empire*, London: Horace Marshall & Son.

Chant, L. (1902) 'Women and the streets', in J. Marchant (ed.) *Public Morals*, London: Morgan and Scott.

Chase, E. (1929) *Tenant Friends in Old Deptford*, London: Williams & Norgate.

CIBA Foundation (1984) *Child Sexual Abuse within the Family*, London: Tavistock.

Clark, A. (1987) 'Womanhood and manhood in the transition from plebeian to working-class culture', PhD thesis, Rutgers University, History Department.

Clarke, J., Cochrane, A. and Smart, C. (1987) *Ideologies of Welfare*, London: Hutchinson.

Collini, S. (1985) 'The idea of "Character" in Victorian political thought', *Transactions of the Royal Historical Society* 35.

Commissioners of Police (1828) *Report*, Parliamentary Papers VI.

Conférence du Code Civil, vols V, XII, Paris: Firmin Didot.

Conrad, H. (1950) 'Die Grundlegung der modernen Zivilehe durch die Französische Revolution', *Zeitschrift der Savigny-Stiftung für Rechtsgeschichte, Germanische Abteilung*, 67: 337–72.

Coole, D. (1988) *Women in Political Theory. From Ancient Misogyny to Contemporary Feminism*, Brighton: Wheatsheaf Books.

Coote, W. (1887) *The Vigilance Record*, 15 April.

Corby, B. (1987) *Working with Child Abuse: Social Work Practice and the Child Abuse System*, Milton Keynes: Open University Press.

Cornwell, J. (1984) *Hard-Earned Lives: Accounts of Health and Illness from East London*, London: Tavistock Publications.

Cott, N. (1979) 'Passionlessness: an interpretation of Victorian sexual ideology, 1790–1851', *Signs* 4: 219–36.

Coward, R. (1983) *Patriarchal Precedents. Sexual and Social Relations*, London: Routledge & Kegan Paul.

Crowther, M.A. (1981) *The Workhouse System 1834–1929*, London: Batsford Academic and Educational Ltd.

Dahl, T.S. and Snare, A. (1978) 'The coercion of privacy', in C. Smart and B. Smart (eds) *Women, Sexuality and Social Control*, London: Routledge & Kegan Paul.

Dale, J. and Foster, P. (1986) *Feminists and State Welfare*, London: Routledge & Kegan Paul.

Darwin, C. (1871) *The Descent of Man*, London.

Davidoff, L. and Hall, C. (1987) *Family Fortunes: Men and Women of the Middle Class*, London: Hutchinson.

Davies, C. (1988) 'The health visitor as mother's friend: a woman's place in public health, 1900–14', *Social History of Medicine* 1 (April).

Davin, A. (1978) 'Imperialism and Motherhood', *History Workshop* 5: 9–65.

Davis, J. (1980) 'The London garotting panic of 1862: a moral panic and the creation of a criminal class in mid-Victorian Britain', in *Crime and the Law: The Social History of Crime in Western Europe since 1500*, London: Europa.

Davis, J. (1984) 'A poor man's system of justice: the London police courts in the second half of the nineteenth century', *Historical Journal*, Vol. 29 (2): 309–33.

De Groot, J. (1989) ' "Sex" and "race": the construction of language and image in the nineteenth century', in S. Mendus and J. Rendall (eds) *Sexuality and Subordination*, London: Routledge.

Dehli, K. (1990) 'An experiment that failed? The Dionne quintuplets as objects of science', unpublished ms, Dept of Sociology of Education, Ontario Institute for Studies in Education.

Delling, G. (1959) 'Ehebruch', *Reallexikon für Antike und Christentum*, vol. 4, cols 666–77, Stuttgart: Anton Hierseman.

Dendy, H. (1893) 'Thorough Charity', *Charity Organisation Review* (June): 204–14.

Dendy, H. (1895a) 'The industrial residuum', in B. Bosanquet (ed.) *Aspects of Social Reform*, London: Macmillan.

Dendy, H. (1895b) 'Marriage in East London', in B. Bosanquet (ed.) *Aspects of Social Reform*, London: Macmillan.

Dendy, H. (1895c) 'The children of working London', in B. Bosanquet (ed.) *Aspects of Social Reform*, London: Macmillan.

Department of Health (1988) *Protecting Children: A Guide for Social Workers Undertaking a Comprehensive Assessment*, London: HMSO.

Department of Health (1989a) *Working with Child Sexual Abuse: Guidelines for Training Social Services Staff*, Child Care Training Support Programme, London: HMSO.

Department of Health (1989b) *An Introduction to the Children Act 1989*, London: HMSO.

Department of Health and Social Security (1988) *Working Together: a Guide to Arrangements for Inter-agency Co-operation for the Protection of Children from Abuse*, London: HMSO.

Derrick, D. (1986) *Illegitimate*, London: National Council for One Parent Families.

Dobash, R.E. and Dobash, R. (1980) *Violence Against Wives*, Somerset: Open Books.

Doggett, M. (1990) 'Wifebeating and the Law in Victorian England', paper presented at the Social Science History Association Conference, Minneapolis.

Donzelot, J. (1979) *The Policing of Families*, London: Hutchinson.

Drucker, W. (1895) 'Vaderschap en Moederschap I, III- VII', *Evolutie* II, 42: 329–31; 43: 337–8; 44: 345–7; 45: 353–4; 46: 361–4; 47: 369–72.

Duby, G. (1988) *Mâle Moyen Age*, Paris: Flammarion.

Eckert, C. (1987) 'Shirley Temple and the House of Rockefeller', in P. Steven (ed.) *Jump-Cut: Hollywood, Politics, Counter-Cinema*, Toronto: Between The Lines.

Edwards, G. (1949) 'Adopting a child', *Quarterly Review* July, 8–13.

Engelstein, L. (1988) 'Gender and the juridical subject: prostitution and rape in nineteenth-century Russian criminal codes', *Journal of Modern History* 60(3): 458–95.

Fairbairn, W.R.D. (1935) 'Medico-psychological aspects of the problem of child assault', *Mental Hygiene* April: 1–16.

Fawcett, J. (1989) 'Breaking the habit: the need for a comprehensive long term treatment for sexually abusing families', in NSPCC, Occasional Paper Series No. 7, *The Treatment of Child Sexual Abuse*, London: NSPCC.

Fawcett, M. (1893) *The Vigilance Record*, June.

Ferguson, H. (1990) 'Rethinking child protection practices: a case for history', in The Violence against Children Study Group, *Taking Child Abuse Seriously*, London: Unwin Hyman.

Fido, J. (1977) 'The charity organisation, society and social casework in London, 1869–1900', in A.P. Donjgrodski (ed.) *Social Control in Nineteenth Century Britain*, London: Croom Helm.

Fielding, E.M. (1953) 'The work of adoption', a report of a conference held at Grove House, Roehampton, July 8–10, convened by the Standing Conference of Societies Registered for Adoption, *Quarterly Review* October.

Finkelhor, D., Hotaling, G. T., Lewis, I.A. and Smith, C. (1990) 'Sexual abuse in a national survey of adult men and women: prevalence, characteristics and risk factors', *Child Abuse & Neglect* 14: 19–28.

Foucault, M (1979) *Discipline and Punish*, New York: Vintage Books.

Foucault, M. (1981) *The History of Sexuality, 1*, Harmondsworth: Pelican.

Fraser, D. (1973) *The Evolution of the Welfare State*, London: Macmillan.

Garland, D. (1985) *Punishment and Welfare: A History of Penal Strategies*, London: Gower.

Gerhard, U. (1978) *Verhältnisse und Verhinderungen. Frauenarbeit, Familie und Rechte der Frauen im Jahrhundert*, Frankfurt: Suhrkamp.

Gerhard, U. (1988) 'Die Rechtsstellung der Frauen in der bürgerlichen Gesellschaft des 19. Jahrhunderts. Frankreich und Deutschland im Vergleich', in J. Kocka (ed.) *Bürgertum im 19. Jahrhundert*, 1, München: Deutscher Taschenbuch Verlag.

Gill, D. (1969) 'Illegitimacy and adoption, its socio-economic correlates, a preliminary report', *Child Adoption* (56): 25–37.

Gillis, J. (1985) *For Better or For Worse: British Marriages 1600 to the Present*, Oxford: Oxford University Press.

Glaser, D. and Spencer, J. R. (1990) 'Sentencing, children's evidence and children's trauma', *Criminal Law Review* June, 371–82.

Gledhill, A. and others (1989) *Who Cares? Children at Risk and Social Services*, London: Centre for Policy Studies.

Gordon, L. (1986) 'Feminism and social control: the case of child abuse and neglect', in J. Mitchell and A. Oakley (eds) *What is Feminism?*, Oxford: Blackwell.

Gordon, L. (1989) *Heroes of their Own Lives: the Politics and History of Family Violence*, London: Virago.

Gordon, L. (1990) Response to Scott, *Signs* 15 (4): 852–3.

Gorham, D. (1978) 'The "Maiden Tribute of Modern Babylon" re-examined: child prostitution and the idea of childhood in late Victorian England', *Victorian Studies* 21 (3): 353–87.

Green, T.A. (1979) Introduction to William Blackstone, *Commentaries on the Laws of England*, 4 vols, Chicago: University of Chicago Press.

Harding, A. (1966) *A Social History of English Law*, Harmondsworth: Penguin.

Harding, S. (1986) *The Science Question in Feminism*, Milton Keynes: Open University Press.

Hawkins, Sir John (1780) *Charge to the Grand Jury of the County of Middlesex*, London.

Hekman, S. (1990) *Gender and Knowledge*, Boston: Northeastern University Press.

Herrup, C. (1990) 'The patriarch at home: the trial of the Earl of Castlehaven for rape and sodomy', paper presented at the Berkshire Conference of Women Historians, June 8–10.

Hill, O. (1869) 'Organised work among the poor, suggestions founded on four years' management of a London court', *Macmillans* 20 (May–October).

Hill, O. (1875) *Homes of the London Poor*, London: Macmillan.

Hill, O. (1888) 'More air for London', *Nineteenth Century* XXIII (January–June).

Hobbes, T. (1651) *Leviathan*, London.

Hoggett, B.M. and Pearl, D. S. (1987) *The Family, Law and Society*, 2nd edn, London: Butterworth.

Hollis, P. (1987) *Ladies Elect. Women in English Local Government, 1865–1914*, Oxford: Clarendon Press.

Holthöfer, E. (1982) 'Frankreich', in H. Coing (ed.) *Handbuch der Quellen and Literatur der Neueren Europäischen Privatrechtsgeschichte*, vol. 3(2), München: Beck.

Hooks, B. (1990) *Yearning: Race, Gender, and Cultural Politics*, Boston: South End Press.

Hooper, C.A. (1990) 'A study of mothers' responses to child sexual abuse by another family member', unpublished PhD thesis, University of London.

Horstman, A. (1985) *Victorian Divorce*, London and Sydney: Croom Helm.

Hostettler, J.A. (1984) 'The curious affair of Lord Cranworth and the criminal law reform in 1853/4', *Anglo- American Law Review* 13 (3): 1–10.

Hume, D. (1965) *Hume's Ethical Writings*, A. MacIntyre (ed.), Paris: University of Notre Dame Press.

Hunt, M. (1988) 'Wifebeating, domesticity, and women's independence in early 18th-century London', paper presented at the American Historical Association meeting, Cincinnati.

Ignatieff, M. (1983) 'Total institutions and working classes: a review essay', *History Workshop Journal* (15): 167–73.

Jansz, U. (1990) *Denken over sekse in de eerste feministische golf*, Amsterdam: Van Gennep.

Jeffreys, S. (1982) ' "Free from all uninvited touch of man": women's campaigns around sexuality, 1880–1914', *Women's Studies International Forum* 5(6): 629–45.

Jeffreys, S. (1985) *The Spinster and Her Enemies*, London: Pandora.

Jeffreys, S. (1989) *Anticlimax, A Feminist Perspective on the Sexual Revolution*, London: The Women's Press Ltd.

Kanthack, E. (1907) *The Preservation of Infant Life*, London: H.K. Lewis.

Kaye, J.M. (1856) Outrages on Women, *North British Review* 25: 256.

Kenny, C.S. (1879) *The History of the Law of England as to the Effect of Marriage on Property and the Wife's Legal Capacity*, London.

Kitzinger, J. (1988) 'Defending innocence: ideologies of childhood', *Feminist Review* 28: 77–87.

Knibiehler, Y. and Fouquet, C. (1983) *La femme et les médecins*, Paris: Hachette.

Kornitzer, M. (1968) *Adoption and Family Life*, London: Putman & Co.

Koven, S. (1987) 'Culture and poverty: The London Settlement House Movement, 1870–1914', unpublished PhD thesis, Harvard University.

Lambertz, J. (1984) 'The politics and economics of family violence, from the late nineteenth century to 1948', M Phil, Manchester University.

Lambertz, J. (1990) 'Feminists and the politics of wifebeating', in H.L. Smith (ed.) *British Feminism in the Twentieth Century*, Boston: University of Massachusetts Press.

Landau, N. (1984) *The Justices of the Peace*, Berkeley: University of California Press.

Laqueur, T. (1987) 'Orgasm, generation, and the politics of reproductive biology', in C. Gallagher and T. Laqueur (eds) *The Making of the Modern Body*, Berkeley: University of California Press.

League of Nations (1934) *Child Welfare Committee Enquiry into the Question of Children in Moral and Social Danger*, Geneva.

Lerner, G. (1986) *The Creation of Patriarchy*, Oxford: Oxford University Press.

Lewis, J. (1980) *The Politics of Motherhood, Child and Maternal Welfare in England, 1900–1939*, London: Croom Helm.

Lewis, J. (1983) *Women's Welfare, Women's Rights*, London: Croom Helm.

Lewis, J. (1984) 'Eleanor Rathbone', in P. Barker (ed.) *Founders of the Welfare State*, London: Gower.

Lewis, J. (1991) *Feminism and Social Problems in the Lives of Five Late Victorian and Edwardian Women*, Cheltenham: Edward Elgar.

Linebaugh, P. (1975) 'The Tyburn riots against the surgeons' in D. Hay, P. Linebaugh, J. Rule, E.P. Thompson and C. Winslow (eds) *Albion's Fatal Tree*, New York: Pantheon.

Locke, J. (1965) *Two Treatises of Government*, London.

Locke, J. (1967) *Two Treatises on Government*, P. Laslett (ed.), Cambridge: Cambridge University Press, 2nd edn.

Lynes, T. (1984) 'William Beveridge 1879–1963', in P. Barker (ed.) *Founders of the Welfare State*, London: Gower.

MacArthur, J.W. and Ford, N. (1937) *A Biological Study of the Dionne Quintuplets: An Identical Set*, Toronto: University of Toronto Press.

McGregor, O.R. (1957) *Divorce in England. A Centenary Study*, London: Heinemann.

McKibbin, R. (1978) 'Social class and social observation in Edwardian England', *Transactions of the Royal Historical Society* 28: 175–200.

McLaren, A. (1978) *Birth Control in Nineteenth Century England*, London: Croom Helm.

MacLeod, M. and Saraga, E. (1988) 'Challenging the orthodoxy: towards a feminist theory and practice', *Feminist Review* 28: 16–55.

MacLeod, V. (1982) *Whose Child? The Family in Child Care, Legislation and Social Work Practice*, London: Study Commission on the Family.

Maine, H.S. (1861) *Ancient Law: its connections with the Early History of Society*, London.

Malcolm, J.P. (1810) *Popular Antiquities*, London.

Manchester, A.H. (1973) 'Simplifying the sources of law: an essay in law reform, part 1: Lord Cranworth's attempt to consolidate the statute law of England and Wales, 1853–9', *Anglo-American Law Review* 2(3): 404–10.

Manvell, R. (1976) *The Trial of Annie Besant*, London: Elek Books.

Martin, A (1911) *Mothers in Mean Streets*, London: United Suffragists.

Masson, J.M. (1985) *The Assault on Truth: Freud's Suppression of the Seduction Theory*, Harmondsworth: Penguin.

Masson, H. and O'Byrne, P. (1990) 'The family systems approach: a help or a hindrance?', in The Violence Against Children Study Group (eds), *Taking Child Abuse Seriously*, London: Unwin Hyman.

Maurice, C.E. (1913) *Life of Octavia Hill*, London: Macmillan.

Maurice, E. (ed.) (1928) *Octavia Hill: Early Ideals*, London: Allen & Unwin.

Maurice, F.D. (1855) *Lectures to Ladies on Practical Subjects*, London: Macmillan.

Maurice, F.D. (1893) *Social Morality*, London: Macmillan.

May, M. (1978) 'Violence in the family: an historical perspective' in J.P. Marton (ed.), *Violence in the Family*, Chicester: John Wiley.

Meek, R.L. (1976) *Social Science and the Ignoble Savage*, Cambridge: Cambridge University Press.

Methuven, M.M. (1948) 'The child, his disadvantages, medical and psychological', Conference paper read at a Symposium on 'The Unmarried Mother and her Child', *Quarterly Review* January: 8–16.

Mill, H.T. (1970) 'The enfranchisement of women', in A. Rossi (ed.) *Essays on Sex Equality: John Stuart Mill and Harriet Taylor*, University of Chicago Press.

Mill, J.S. (1869) *The Subjection of Women*, London.

Mitchell, H. (1968) *The Hard Way Up*, London: Virago.

Mitra, C. (1987) 'Judicial discourse in father-daughter incest appeal cases', *International Journal of the Sociology of Law* 15(2): 121–48.

Moral Reform Union (n.d.) *The Fallen Woman!* (leaflet).

Mort, F. (1987) *Dangerous Sexualities: Medico-Moral Politics in England since 1830*, London: Routledge & Kegan Paul.

Mowat, C.L. (1961) *The Charity Organisation Society, 1869–1913*, London: Methuen.

National Association for Mental Health (1953) *Memorandum on Adoption for Home Office Adoption of Children Committee*, London.

National Council for the Unmarried Mother and her Child (NCUMC) (1968) *The Human Rights of Those Born Out of Wedlock*, 50 Golden Jubilee, London: NCUMC.

Nead, L. (1988) *Myths of Sexuality*, Oxford: Blackwell.

Nelson, S. (1987) *Incest: Fact and Myth*, Edinburgh: Stramullion Press.

Nevinson, M.W. (1926) *Life's Fitful Fever*, London: A&C Black.

Nimey, J. (1986) *Time of their Lives*, Ottawa: Nivan.

Norton, C. (1978) 'English laws for women', in *Selected Writings of Caroline Norton*, Delmar, New York: Scholars Facsimilies and Reprints.

O'Hagan, K. (1989) *Working with Child Sexual Abuse*, Milton Keynes: Open University Press.

Orkin, M. (1981) *The Great Stork Derby*, Toronto: General.

Pahl, J. (1980) 'Patterns of money management within marriage', *Journal of Social Policy* 9(3).

Pahl, J. (1985) *Private Violence and Public Policy: The Needs of Battered Women and the Response of the Public Services*, London: Routledge & Kegan Paul.

Pateman, C. (1989) *The Sexual Contract*, Stanford, California: Stanford University Press.

Pearsall, R. (1975) *Night's Black Angels*, London: Hodder & Stoughton.

Pennybacker, S. (1986) 'It was not what she said but the way in which she said it', in P. Bailey (ed.) *Music Hall: the Business of Pleasure*, Oxford: Oxford University Press.

Phillips, R. (1980) *Family Breakdown in Late Eighteenth Century France*, Oxford: Clarendon Press.

Pinkerton, M.W. (1898) *Murder in All Ages*, Chicago: Pinkerton & Co.

Pithouse, A. (1987) *Social Work: the Social Organisation of an Invisible Trade*, Aldershot: Avebury.

Pleck, E. (1987) *Domestic Tyranny: The Making of American Social Policy against Family Violence from Colonial Times to the Present*, Oxford: Oxford University Press.

Pochin, J. (1969) *Without a Wedding Ring: Casework with Unmarried Parents* (introduction by Pauline Shapiro), London: Constable.

Portemer, J. (1962) 'Le Statut de la Femme en France Depuis la Réformation des Coûtumes Jusqu'à la Rédaction du Code Civil', *Recueils de la Société Jean Bodin* 12(2), 444–97.

Poovey, M. (1989) *Uneven Developments*, London: Virago.

Prochaska, F. (1980) *Women and Philanthropy in Nineteenth Century England*, Oxford: Clarendon.

Prochaska, F. (1988) *The Voluntary Impulse, Philanthropy in Modern Britain*, London: Faber & Faber.

Radzinowicz, Sir L. (1948) *A History of the English Criminal Law*, London: Stevens, 4 vols.

Rendall, J. (1987) 'Virtue and commerce: women in the making of Adam Smith's political economy', in E. Kennedy and S. Mendus (eds) *Women in Western Political Philosophy*, Brighton: Wheatsheaf Books.

Report of the Care of Children Committee (Chaired by Lady Curtis) (1946) (Curtis Report), London: HMSO.

Report of the Departmental Committee on Sexual Offences against Young Persons (1925) London: HMSO.

Report of the Royal Commission on the Housing of the Working classes (1885) Vol II, Minutes of Evidence, C. 4402–1, London: HMSO.

Returns relating to Assaults on Women and Children, from Each of the Metropolitan Police Courts, 1854–1855, Parliamentary Papers, LIII.

Rich, A. (1977) *Of Woman Born: Motherhood as Experience and Institution*, London: Virago.

Riley, D. (1979) 'War in the Nursery', *Feminist Review* (2).

Riley, D. (1983) *War in the Nursery*, London: Virago.

Riley, D. (1988) *'Am I that Name?' Feminism and the Category of 'Woman' in History*, London: Macmillan.

Roberts, E. (1984) *A Woman's Place, An Oral History of Working-Class Women 1890–1940*, Oxford: Blackwell.

Roberts, M.J.D. (1985) 'Morals, art and the law: The Obscene Publications Act of 1852', *Victorian Studies* 28(4): 609–30.

Roberts, S. (1983) 'The study of disputes: anthropological perspectives', in J. Bossy (ed.) *Disputes and Settlements*, Cambridge: Cambridge University Press.

Rose, M.E. (1971) *The English Poor-Law 1780–1930*, London: David & Charles.

Ross, E. (1983) ' "Fierce Questions and Taunts": married life in working-class London, 1870–1914', *Feminist Studies* 8(3): 575–602.

Rowbotham, S. (1973) *Hidden from History*, London: Pluto Press.

Rush, F. (1984) 'The Freudian cover-up', *Trouble & Strife* 4: 29–36.

Russell, D. (1984) *Sexual Exploitation: Rape, Child Sexual Abuse and Workplace Harassment*, London: Sage.

Russell, W.O. (1819) *A Treatise on Crimes and Misdemeanours*, London, 2 vols.

Sagnac, P. (1898) *La Législation Civile de la Révolution Française (1798–1804)*, Paris: Librairie Hachette et C.

Sauer, R. (1978) 'Infanticide and abortion in nineteenth-century Britain', *Population Studies* 32(1): 81–93.

Savigny, D.F. von (1845) 'Revision des Strafgesetzbuches von 1843', in Gerhard, *Verhältnisse* (1978), 451–2.

Savigny, D.F. von (1850) 'Darstellung der in den Preussischen Gesetzen-über die Ehescheidung unternommenen Reform', in Savigny, *Vermischte Schriften*, Vol. 5, Aalen: Scientia Verlag, 222–343.

Schleifer, C.H. (1972) 'Die Ehescheidung im deutschen Rechtskreis', doctoral dissertation, University of Kiell.

Schnapper, B. (1987) 'Autorité domestique et partis politiques de Napoléonà de Gaulle', in H. Mohnhaput (ed.) *Zur Geschichte des Familien-und Erbrechts*, Frankfurt: Vittorio Klostermann.

Scott, A.F. (1984) 'On seeing and not seeing: a case of historical invisibility', *Journal of American History* 71.

Scott, J. (1990) Review of Linda Gordon, *Heroes of Their Own Lives: the Politics and History of Family Violence*, *Signs* 15(4): 848–52.

Sevenhuijsen, S.L. (1987) *De orde van het vaderschap. Politieke debatten over afstamming, huwelijk en ongehuwd moederschap in Nederland 1870–1900*, Amsterdam: IISG Beheer.

Sharpe, J.A. (1983) *Crime in Seventeenth Century England*, Cambridge: Cambridge University Press.

Shaw, L.A. (1953) 'Following up adoptions', *British Journal of Psychiatric Social Work*, May (6): 14–21.

Shuttleworth, S. (1990) 'Female circulation: medical discourse and popular advertising in the mid-Victorian era', in M. Jacobus, E. Fox Keller and S Shuttleworth (eds) *Body/Politics*, London: Routledge.

Simpson, A. (1984) *Biographical Dictionary of the Common Law*, London: Butterworth.

Sinha, M. (1987) 'Gender and imperialism: colonial policy and the ideology of moral imperialism in late nineteenth-century Bengal', in M. Kimmel (ed.) *Changing Men*, London: Sage.

Smart, C. (1982) 'Regulating families or legitimating patriarchy', *International Journal of the Sociology of Law*, 10(2): 129–47.

Smart C. (1984) *The Ties that Bind*, London: Routledge & Kegan Paul.

Smart, C. (1989) *Feminism and the Power of the Law*, London: Routledge.

Smith, A. (1978) *Lectures on Jurisprudence*, in R.L. Meek, D.D. Raphael and P.G. Stein (eds), Oxford: Oxford University Press.

Spelman, E.V. (1982) 'Woman as body: ancient and contemporary views', *Feminist Studies* 8 (1): 109–31.

Spelman, E.V. (1988) *Inessential Woman*, Boston: Beacon Press.

Spensky, M. (1988) 'La prise en charge des mères célibataires et de leurs enfants en Angleterre: 19ème et 20ème siècles', unpublished PhD Thesis, Université de Paris, VIII.

Stark, E. and Flitcraft, A. (1988) 'Women and children at risk: a feminist perspective on child abuse', *International Journal of Health Services* 18(1): 97–118.

Staves, S. (1990) *Married Women and Property in England, 1660–1823*, Boston: Harvard University Press.

Stedman Jones, G. (1976) *Outcast London*, Harmondsworth: Penguin.

Stedman Jones, G. (1977) 'Class expression vs. Social control. A critique of recent trends in the social history of "leisure" ', *History Workshop Journal* 4: 162–70.

Stein, P. (1980) *Legal Evolution. The Story of an Idea*, Cambridge: Cambridge University Press.

Steinmetz, S.R. (1895) 'Verheffing en bevrijding der vrouw', in F.R. Lapidoth (ed.) *Los en Vast*, 314–330.

Steinmetz, S.R. (1896) 'Verheffing en bevrijding der vrouw', in F.R. Lapidoth, (ed.) *Los en Vast*, 46–8, 187–202, 245–79, 314–30, 335–75, 375–93.

Strong-Boag, V. (1988) *The New Day Recalled: Lives of Girls and Women in English Canada 1919–1939*, Toronto: Copp Clark Pitman.

Summerfield, P. (1981) 'The Effingham Arms and the Empire', in E. Yeo and S. Yeo (eds) *Popular Culture and Class Conflict, 1590–1914*, Brighton: Harvester Press.

Summerfield, P. (1984) *Women Workers in the Second World War*, London: Croom Helm.

Summers, A. (1979) 'A home from home: women's philanthropic work in the nineteenth century', in S. Burman (ed.) *Fit Work for Women*, London: Croom Helm.

Sutherland, N. (1976) *Children in English Canadian Society: Creating the Twentieth Century Consensus*, Toronto: University of Toronto Press.

Tebbut, M. (1983) *Making Ends Meet, Pawnbroking and Working Class Credit*, Leicester: Leicester University Press.

Teichman, J. (1982) *Illegitimacy, An Examination of Bastardy*, New York: Cornell University Press.

Thane, P. (1984) 'The working class and state "welfare" in Britain, 1880–1914', *Historical Journal* 27.

The Annual Register (1835) or *A view of the History, Politics and Literature of the Year 1834*, London: Baldwin & Cradock, Chapter VI: 222.

Thomas, K. (1959) 'The Double Standard', *Journal of the History of Ideas* 20: 195–216.

Thompson, E.P. (1972) ' "Rough music": le Charivari anglais', *Annales: ESC* 27(2): 286–312.

Thompson, E.P. (1975) *Whigs and Hunters: The Origins of the Black Acts*, New York: Pantheon.

Thompson, F.M.L. (1981) 'Social control in Victorian Britain', *Economic History Review* XXXIV, May: 189–208.

Titmuss, R. (1950) *Problems of Social Policy*, London: HMSO.

Tomes, N. (1978) ' "A Torrent of Abuse": crimes of violence between working-class men and women in London, 1840–1875', *Journal of Social History* 11: 238–345.

Townsend, W.C. (1846) *Lives of Twelve Eminent Judges*, London.

Traer, J.F. (1980) *Marriage and Family in Eighteenth-Century France*, Ithaca and London: Cornell University Press.

Truesdell, D.J., McNeil, J.S. and Deschner, J.P. (1986) 'Incidence of wife abuse in incestuous families', *Social Work* Mar–Apr: 138–40.

Underdown, D. (1985) 'The taming of the scold: the enforcement of patriarchal authority in early modern England', in A. Fletcher and J. Stevenson (eds) *Order and Disorder in Early Modern England*, Cambridge: Cambridge University Press.

Valverde, M. (1990) 'The rhetoric of reform: tropes and the moral subject' *International Journal of the Sociology of Law* 18: 1.

Valverde, M. (1991) *'The Age of Light, Soap, and Water'*: *Moral Reform in English Canada 1880s-1920s*, Toronto: McClelland & Stewart.

Vicinus, M. (1986) *Independent Women*, London: Virago Press.

Vincent, A.W. (1984) 'The Poor Law Reports of 1909 and the social theory of the COS', *Victorian Studies* (Spring) 27: 343–63.

Vincent, A. and Plant, R. (1984) *Philosophy, Politics and Citizenship*, Oxford: Blackwell.

Vogel, U (1986) 'Rationalism and romanticism: two strategies for women's emancipation', in J. Evans, J. Hills, K. Hunt, E. Meehan, T. ten Tusschon, U. Vogel and G. Waylen (eds) *Feminism and Political Theory*, London: Sage.

Vogel, U. (1988) 'Patriarchale Herrschaft, bürgerliches Recht, bürgerliche Utopie. Eigentumsrechte der Frauen in Deutschland und England', in J. Kocka (ed.) *Bürgertum im 19. Jahrhundert*, vol. 1, München: Deutscher Taschenbuch Verlag.

Vogel, U. (1990) 'Eve and the Amazon: conflicting images of gender in natural law', paper presented at the International Symposium on Law, Morality and Virtue in the Enlightenment, Amsterdam.

Vogeli, W. (1988) 'Funktionswandel des Scheidungsrechts', *Kritische Justiz* 7.

Walby, S. (1990) 'From private to public patriarchy: the periodisation of British history', *Women's Studies International Forum*, 13 (1/2): 91–104.

Walkowitz, J. (1984) 'Male vice and female virtue: feminism and the politics of prostitution in nineteenth-century Britain', in A. Snitow, C. Stansell and S. Thompson (eds) *Desire: The Politics of Sexuality*, London: Virago.

Weedon, C. (1987) *Feminist Practice and Poststructuralist Theory*, Oxford: Blackwell.

Weeks, J. (1989) *Sex, Politics and Society*, London: Longman, 2nd edn.

Wharton, J.J.S. (1853) *An Exposition of the Law relating to the Women of England, Showing Their Rights, Remedies and Responsibilities in Every Position of Law*, London.

Wijnaendts Francken (1894) *De evolutie van het huwelijk. Eene sociologische studie*, Leiden.

Wijnaendts Francken (1896) *De vrouwenbeweging*, Haarlem.

Williams, R. (1983) *Keywords: A Vocabulary of Culture and Society*, New York: Oxford University Press.

Wilson, E. (1977) *Women and the Welfare State*, London: Tavistock Publications.

Wilson, E. (1980) *Only Half-Way to Paradise, Women in Post-war Britain: 1945-1968*, London: Tavistock Publications

Wilson, L. (1886) 'Editorial', *Personal Rights Journal* 15 January.

Wohl, A. (1971) 'Octavia Hill and the homes of the London Poor', *Journal of British Studies*, 10 (May).

Wohl, A.S. (1978), 'Sex and the single room: incest among the Victorian working classes', in A.S. Wohl (ed.) *The Victorian Family*, London: Croom Helm.

Wolf, S.C., Conte, J.R. and Engel-Meinig, M. (1988) 'Assessment and treatment of sex offenders in a community setting', in L. Walker (ed.), *Handbook on Sexual Abuse of Children*, New York: Springer.

Wolstenholme Elmy, E. (1886a) *Journal of the Personal Rights Association*, March.

Wolstenholme Elmy, E. (1886b) *Journal of the Personal Rights Association*, May.

Wolstenholme Elmy, E. (1887) *Journal of the Personal Rights Association*, May.

Wood, N. (1982) 'Prostitution and feminism in nineteenth-century Britain' *m/f* no. 7.

Woodroofe, K. (1974) *From Charity to Social Work*, London: Routledge & Kegan Paul.

Young, L. (1954) *Out of Wedlock*, New York: McGraw-Hill Book Company.

Index